THE
CLEAR
–SKIN–
PROTOCOL

TREAT THE ROOT
CAUSES OF ACNE

. . . .

RENELLE STAYTON
FNP-BC

This book is intended to supplement, not replace, the advice of a trained health professional. If you know or suspect that you have a health problem, you should consult a health professional before embarking on any medical program or treatment. The author disclaims any liability for any medical outcomes that may occur as a result of applying the methods suggested in this book.

First edition: October 2020

Renelle Stayton website: www.RenelleStayton.com

Ebook ISBN: 978-1-7353727-0-9
Print ISBN: 978-1-7353727-3-0

TABLE OF CONTENTS

*For Jeremy, whose insight, encouragement,
love and recipes made this book possible*

INTRODUCTION

You have acne. And you're out of options.

You've used antibiotics, birth control pills, benzoyl peroxide and retinoids. You've tried all of the over-the-counter acne products, your friend's apple cider vinegar cleanse and the 15-step skincare regimen you found on r/skincareaddiction.

Nothing works.

In fact, your skin seems to be getting worse rather than better. You thought that by the time you were 20—or 25, or even 35—your acne would have magically disappeared. That's the way it's supposed to work: clear skin after your teenage years, no more worrying about breakouts. Yet, here you are...and your skin is worse than ever.

If this sounds familiar, *then this book is for you.*

If you follow the protocol, your skin will get better and it will stay better. No more worrying when the ball is going to drop, or that you're late to pick up a prescription. No more rush deliveries of products that you ran out of.

Imagine feeling relaxed about your skin. Or not even thinking about it at all.

Clear skin is possible without a prescription.

I won't lie to you and say that it's going to be a walk in the park.

It's going to take a lot of preparation, time and self-control. But once you have the right tools, you'll be able to maintain clear skin for the rest of your life.

You can do this!

I'm here to help you every step of the way. I wouldn't ask you to do any of these things if I didn't think you were capable (and if I hadn't already done them myself).

Here's what you'll learn from this book

- Why you have acne

- Why conventional treatments don't work

- What the root causes of acne are

- Why healing your gut is key to healing your skin

- How to identify your gut imbalance

- How to follow a therapeutic food and supplement plan to fix your gut issue

- What foods heal acne

- What supplements restore skin and gut health

- Which natural therapies should be included in your skincare routine

- How to design your lifestyle to support radiant skin and overall health

What you won't learn

- **The quick fix for acne.** Healing takes time, especially if there are more severe imbalances involved.

- **How to get clear skin without making some big changes to your diet and lifestyle.** I'll be asking you to follow a very specific food plan which takes time to adapt to if you're not used to grocery shopping, meal planning or cooking for yourself.

- **The "one-size-fits-all" diet for acne.** What may be therapeutic for one person may not work at all for another. Diet should be tailored to meet the individual needs of the person.

- **The strict vegan diet for acne.** While plant-based foods are an integral part of each of the food plans, many of the therapeutic foods for acne and recipes in this book are not plant-based. You will need to make appropriate substitutions as you see fit.

- **A 10-step skincare routine.** Too many products with too many ingredients can make breakouts worse.

This might sound harsh, but I don't want to waste your time. Keep reading if you think that this still sounds like a good fit.

WHY SHOULD YOU TAKE MY ADVICE?

Hi, I'm Renelle. I'm a family nurse practitioner who specializes in functional medicine, as well as a certified holistic nutritionist.

Despite my training and work experience in conventional medicine, it failed me when it came to treating my acne.

I had severe acne for over a decade and spent thousands of dollars on acne treatments that never fixed the underlying problem. My skin continued to get worse as I got older, despite using multiple rounds of antibiotics, birth control pills, retinoids, benzoyl peroxide, salicylic acid, etc.

By the time I was 22, my face was broken out all of the time and none of my medications were working. At this point, I knew something needed to change. I decided to take my health into my own hands and began to experiment with alternative acne treatments.

It wasn't a quick fix. I failed *a lot* before figuring out what worked.

At times, it felt like I was stuck in a never-ending cycle of trial and error. I'd break out, start using something new, have clear skin for awhile, then I'd break out again. Sometimes I'd go back to using medications and they would still not work. This cycle would continue until I was almost 30.

Here's what I tried:

- Paleo diet
- GAPS diet
- Ketogenic diet
- Cleansing my face with dandruff shampoo
- Sulfur ointment
- Probiotic enemas
- Regular facials with an esthetician
- Acupuncture
- Traditional Chinese medicine herbs
- Oil cleansing with coconut oil

- Ayurvedic herbs
- And many others...

Every time something would fail, I was devastated.

It was heartbreaking to wake up day after day with a face full of new pimples and no end in sight. Taking off my makeup and looking at my bare skin would make me want to burst into tears. People would suggest things I should try for my skin, which would only make me feel humiliated and depressed.

Despite how awful this time was, it motivated me to figure out a solution. I refused to believe that acne was something I was going to have to get used to having forever.

At 26, after working for several years in the pediatric and neo-natal intensive care units as a nurse, I applied to graduate school to become a nurse practitioner. I also began training in functional medicine and holistic nutrition.

By 29, I'd applied what I'd learned to myself. I treated my SIBO and leaky gut, corrected my nutrient deficiencies, stopped taking antibiotics and hormonal birth control pills, simplified my skincare routine, switched to natural skincare products and over-hauled my lifestyle to improve my health.

And guess what? My skin got clear and stayed clear. **And it's still clear today.**

I became that person who didn't give their skin a second thought when they woke up in the morning (something I'd always dreamed of!). I stopped wearing makeup. I didn't obsess over how my skin looked under horrible fluorescent lighting. I received compliments on my skin for the first time ever.

I had found the holy grail: clear skin without a prescription.

It was a bumpy road (haha) but there were some valuable take-aways:

- **I had to take my health into my own hands and become my own health detective.** I became my own science experiment, researching and trying out different kinds of diets, herbs, products, cleanses, etc. I also expanded my education to learn how to approach health from a holistic perspective.

- **Conventional medicine didn't have all of the answers and I couldn't rely on medications.** The long-term solution for my acne had always been to suppress it with medications. I remember going to my first dermatologist appointment when I was 14. I was prescribed oral antibiotics and a variety of topical medications, which I continued using, on and off, for almost 10 years. When these failed, it reinforced the idea that the conventional approach was not going to fix my problem.

- **Functional medicine and holistic nutritionist training provided a framework that made sense.** While I was fortunate to be trained as a nurse prac-titioner at a top-ranked university, what I learned in functional medicine and holistic nutritionist training was more impactful. As I continued to go down the less conventional path, I began to see health in a com-pletely different way. Rather than view the body as an isolated set of organ systems, I saw how integrated and interconnected everything was. I learned how to view health from a whole-body, personalized perspective. I discovered the healing power of food and how the gastrointestinal, immune and endocrine systems impacted skin health.

It took me a long time to figure out how to work *with* my body instead of against it. I wrote this book to prevent you from having to go through the same struggles that I did. My mission is to give you the tools to clear your skin and maintain it for the rest of your life.

Let's get started.

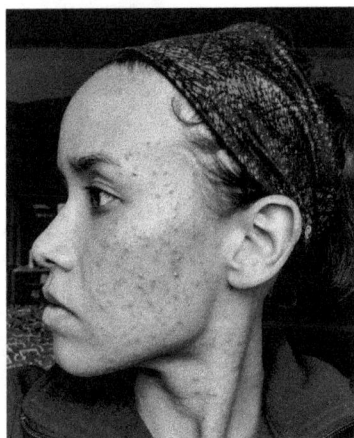

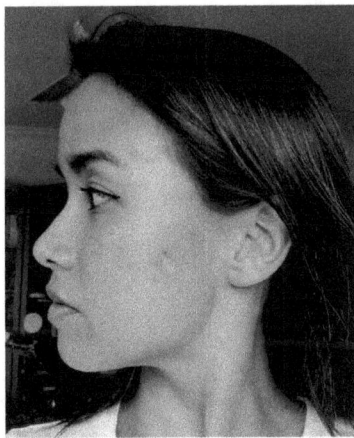

I've included a summary and key takeaways at the end of each chapter. To jump straight to the protocol, go to Chapter 3. You can also refer to the Cheat Sheet at the end of the book.

CHAPTER 1

WHAT IS FUNCTIONAL MEDICINE?

"If you are sitting on a tack, the answer is not to treat the pain. The solution is to find the tack and remove it."

—SIDNEY BAKER, MD

Functional medicine is evidence-based, personalized medicine that doesn't rely on medications alone to restore health. It treats the root cause of disease, rather than suppress symptoms, in order to restore balance and function.

While conventional medicine wants to figure out "what" disease you have, functional medicine wants to figure out "why" you have it in the first place.

Let me be clear that conventional medicine is unbeatable when it comes to fixing acute or life-threatening problems, like breaking your arm or suffering a traumatic brain injury. However, its heavy-hitting approach isn't suited to manage many chronic diseases in primary care.

Functional medicine enhances the conventional approach, it doesn't reject it. Providers are still informed by the same standard-of-care practices and will use medications if medically indicated. However, functional medicine uses other tools to assess and optimize your state of health that make its treatment approach more personalized, effective and sustainable.

If you visit a functional medicine provider, you'll spend 1-2 hours reviewing your health history and primary concerns. This allows your provider to get a thorough understanding of what events have set the stage for your current state of health.

You may be asked to provide a food diary for nutritional analysis, a stool sample to evaluate your microbiome, genetic testing to look at any factors that can affect your ability to detoxify, or a number of other tests that provide a better understanding of your health.

Your provider can help you identify the major imbalances that are contributing to your health problem, working with you to create a personalized treatment plan. Treatment will often include an intensive therapeutic food plan, targeted supplement therapy and other lifestyle interventions to optimize health.

SUMMARY

Conventional medicine wants to know "what" disease you have while functional medicine wants to know "why" you have it in the first place.

Gathering a detailed health history helps your functional medicine provider identify what potential imbalances are contributing to your health concern. There are diagnostic tools that these providers utilize that are not routinely used in conventional medicine. Most treatment plans are centered around a therapeutic diet, supplement regimen and lifestyle interventions.

Key takeaways

- Functional medicine is evidence-based, personalized medicine that doesn't rely on medications alone to restore health
- Treating the root cause of disease is key for restoring health and balance to your body

CHAPTER 2

WHY YOU HAVE ACNE

"It's more important to understand the imbalances in your body's basic systems and restore balance, rather than name the disease and match the pill to the ill."

—MARK HYMAN, MD

Acne is a symptom of an underlying imbalance in one or more of your body systems: your gut, your immune system, your endocrine (hormone) system or your mind-body connection.

But what causes imbalance in the first place?

The answer is inflammation, oxidative stress and hormone imbalance—the root causes of acne.

While conventional acne treatments treat the bacteria or excess sebum (oil) that contribute to acne, they don't treat what causes the changes in the skin in the first place. The good news is that you *can* treat the underlying root causes. As you'll learn in this chapter, most of them are modifiable with diet, supplements and lifestyle interventions.

INFLAMMATION

Inflammation underlies most chronic diseases, including: arthritis, cancer, eczema, type 2 diabetes, obesity, cardiovascular disease, depression and neurodegenerative disorders [1-5].

Acne is no exception [6-8].

Inflammation is the body's normal response to injury and is beneficial in small amounts for short amounts of time. Redness, swelling, pain and heat are all signs of inflammation. They signal your immune system to repair damaged tissue and also help protect against invasion by foreign pathogens.

When inflammation becomes chronic, it can promote disease. **For skin issues like acne, the source of chronic inflammation is usually the gut.**

Let's take a closer look at factors that worsen inflammation: sugar and dairy, nutrient deficiencies, leaky gut, food sensitivities and allergies, gut imbalances and infections, toxins and stress.

Sugar and dairy

Sugar and dairy cause inflammation and hormone imbalances that contribute to acne.

The problem with eating too much sugar is that it increases blood sugar and insulin levels too much [9-14].

How does this relate to the skin?

When you eat foods high in sugar, your blood sugar level rises quickly. Your pancreas then pumps out a hormone called insulin, which transports the blood sugar into cells. High insulin levels increase androgens (also known as "male sex hormones") which stimulate sebum production, promote inflammation and cause overproduction of skin cells.

High Sugar Foods

- Artificial and natural sweeteners
- Dried fruit
- Flavored coffee drinks
- Granola
- Low-fat yogurt
- Processed junk food
- Protein bars
- Starches
- Sugary beverages (fruit juice, sports drinks, energy drinks, iced tea, soda)
- White flour products (bagels, bread, pasta)

Dairy isn't much better. Milk and other dairy products contain cow reproductive hormones, inflammatory proteins (casein and whey) and growth factors. These are meant to help baby cows grow—they're not doing your skin any favors [15,16]. They're bad for your skin because they overstimulate your growth hormone systems.

Dairy increases insulin levels as much as sugar does [16-18]. This is due to the whey protein found in milk. Whey proteins also contain betacellulin, a growth factor that binds to receptors on skin cells, telling them to multiply. Casein raises IGF-1 (insulin-like growth factor) levels which increases androgens and stimulates overproduction of sebum and skin cells [18,19]. This leads to clogged pores and acne.

Nutrient deficiencies

When you're deficient in certain nutrients, like zinc or omega 3s, it's harder for your body to fight inflammation and heal your skin. In today's world, it's difficult to get enough nutrients from food alone. This is due to factors like nutrient-depleted soil and increasing use of genetically modified foods.

Leaky gut

Leaky gut plays a major role in acne [20]. It's a condition where your gut barrier becomes more permeable (or "leaky") to substances that would normally not be allowed through.

In other words, your gut barrier becomes like Swiss cheese.

HEALTHY GUT   **LEAKY GUT**

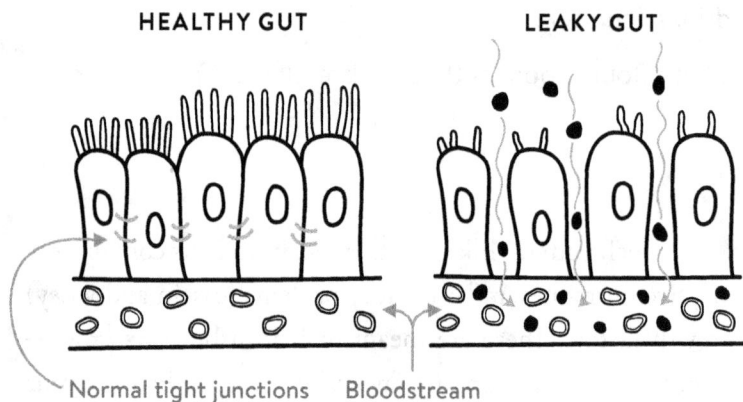

Normal tight junctions   Bloodstream

This is problematic because partially digested food particles, bacteria, yeast and chemicals can leak into your bloodstream and activate your immune system. Your immune system—which doesn't recognize these foreign substances—sets off an alarm to the rest of your body, causing inflammation and even autoimmune disorders in some cases [21]. Leaky gut can also predispose you to developing food sensitivities.

The Immune System in Your Gut

Did you know that 80% of your immune system is in your gut? It's called the gut-associated lymphoid tissue (GALT). Since your gut is one of your body's largest interfaces with the outside world, it's understandable why such a big part of your immune system lives there.

Causes of leaky gut

- Food sensitivities and allergies
- Gluten [22,23]
- Alcohol
- Birth control pills
- Drugs like antibiotics and NSAIDs (Advil, Motrin)
- Low stomach acid (use of acid-blocking drugs)
- Gut imbalances (Candida overgrowth, SIBO)
- Chronic stress [24]

Food sensitivities and allergies

Unlike food allergies, which cause an immediate and severe immune reaction, food sensitivities cause reactions that are delayed, often by hours or even days.

Common food sensitivities are: dairy, gluten, eggs, corn, soy and peanuts. Reactions can vary from person to person depending on the food being eaten, but common reactions include: acne, brain fog, eczema, fatigue, joint pain, runny nose, headache or difficulty sleeping.

Gut imbalances and infections

Gut imbalances like yeast overgrowth (also referred to as Candida) and small intestinal bacterial overgrowth (SIBO) are common, especially if you have acne. You'll assess which imbalance you may be dealing with in Chapter 5.

Gut infections are also a source of chronic inflammation. Stool testing may be required to identify more insidious infections, caused by things like parasites or worms.

Toxins

Your ability to get rid of toxins depends on your organs of elimination: your gut, liver, kidneys and skin. When you're exposed to toxins in everyday life—through the environment, drugs, food, personal care products—this increases what's known as your "toxic burden". You want your toxic burden to be low so that your detoxification organs can manage the toxins properly. If your toxic burden is too high, your systems can get overwhelmed, leading to chronic inflammation, dysfunction and disease.

The Bucket Analogy

Imagine your body as an empty bucket starting at the time you were born. As you're exposed to toxins in everyday life, drops of water go into the bucket. If your bucket fills up too quickly, it will overflow, causing health problems. Minimize the amount of water that goes into your bucket.

Stress

While short periods of stress can be beneficial, chronic stress wreaks havoc on your body. Stress hormones, like cortisol and adrenaline, are meant to be used if there is an immediate threat to your physical safety. They give you quick energy to escape imminent danger, but if they're chronically elevated, they cause cellular inflammation, insulin resistance, weight gain, decreased secretory IgA in your gut (which protects your gut barrier) and weakened immune function. Important skin healing nutrients, like vitamin C and zinc, are also depleted by chronic stress.

Your body can't tell the difference between real stress—like running from a bear—and perceived stress—like running late for work. So just *thinking* that you're under stress has the same hormonal effect as running away from a bear.

OXIDATIVE STRESS

Like inflammation, oxidative stress underlies many chronic diseases, including: heart disease, type 2 diabetes, autoimmune disorders and chronic obstructive pulmonary disease [25-29]. People with acne have higher levels of oxidative stress markers compared to healthy controls [30,31].

What is oxidative stress? It refers to an imbalance between the amount of free radicals in your body and the amount of antioxidants that are available to neutralize them. Free radicals are generated as a normal byproduct of metabolism in your cells. They're missing an electron, so they travel throughout your system to find cells that they can scavenge electrons from. The cells that they steal electrons from are left damaged, and the damaged cells then have to go find electrons to bring them back to stability. **If you don't have enough antioxidants to regularly counteract free radical damage, over time, your body won't be able to repair itself.**

Next you'll look at the factors that increase oxidative stress: not enough antioxidants, smoking, drugs, toxins and poor sleep.

Not enough antioxidants

Not getting enough antioxidants from your diet is a major contributor to oxidative stress. If your diet is lacking in fresh fruits and vegetables, you're more likely to be deficient.

Smoking

Smoking releases free radicals and thousands of different chemicals into your body. It also makes acne worse: nicotine increases sebum retention and scaling within the follicles, which causes whiteheads and blackheads.

Drugs

Overuse of acetaminophen (Tylenol) depletes glutathione, which is a crucial antioxidant. Other drugs generate high levels of oxidative stress as they're metabolized, like non-steroidal anti-inflammatory drugs (NSAIDs), antipsychotics, antiretrovirals and certain cancer therapies.

Toxins

Exposure to environmental toxins is a major source of oxidative stress. Things like pollution and mold exhaust antioxidant stores. Pesticides found on conventional produce deplete cellular energy, making it difficult for cells to fight free radicals. Heavy metals, such as those found in dental amalgam fillings, interfere with the antioxidant glutathione.

Poor sleep

Your body repairs itself while you sleep. When you don't sleep enough, it inhibits skin healing and increases markers of oxidative stress [32].

HORMONE IMBALANCE

Hormones are chemical messengers that travel to specific bodily tissues and affect how they function. There are several hormones that can be associated with acne, including: testosterone, estrogen, progesterone, cortisol and insulin. How these hormones work together and their specific ratios relative to one another can affect your skin. If one is off—too high, or too low—it can throw the others off, too.

Rather than focus on *what* hormones are causing the problem, it's important to figure out *why* they're out of balance in the first place.

So, first you'll look at the *why*, and then I'll briefly discuss two types of hormone imbalances that are associated with acne.

Sugar and dairy

These foods and their hormonal impact were already covered in the beginning of this chapter. The bottom line is that they both increase insulin levels, which triggers a cascade that leads to breakouts.

Hormonal birth control pills

The pill negatively affects hormone, gut and skin health. This is not routinely discussed with women when they're first prescribed it. While this could be an entire book on its own, the bottom line is that **I do not recommend the pill for acne or as a birth control method.**

When you take the pill, it floods your body with synthetic hormones that shut off the delicate communication between your brain and ovaries. It doesn't fix the problem of bad skin or painful periods…it only masks the problem.

The pill causes nutrient deficiencies (like zinc deficiency) that make acne worse. It also increases the likelihood that you'll develop leaky gut or Candida overgrowth and worsens gut inflammation. After you stop taking the pill, it can cause a rebound in testosterone levels which can lead to bad breakouts.

To learn more about the effects of the pill and transitioning off of it, read *Beyond the Pill* by naturopathic doctor Jolene Brighten.

Hormone disrupting toxins

These are also known as "endocrine disruptors." They mimic real hormones and prevent real hormones from doing their job. They've been associated with many adverse health effects, including: impaired immune function, diabetes, learning disabilities and obesity.

Examples of endocrine disruptors:

- Phthalates - found in fragrances and plastic food containers
- Pesticides - found on non-organic produce
- Triclosan - found in antibacterial soaps

- Perfluorochemicals - found in non-stick pans, micro-wave popcorn bags and clothing
- Xenoestrogens - found in personal care products, pesticides, certain plastics, BPA

Poor detoxification

When your detoxification organs aren't working properly this means that hormones that were meant to get eliminated get reabsorbed and recirculated through your body. These are usually more potent and harmful forms of these hormones.

For example, constipation (<1 bowel movement daily) is a sign of impaired detoxification. If you're not eliminating regularly through pooping, your skin becomes one of the default organs to get rid of toxins, which can make breakouts even worse.

HORMONE IMBALANCE 1: ESTROGEN DOMINANCE

This condition occurs when there is too much estrogen relative to progesterone or just too much estrogen, period. When estrogen levels are too high, it can have widespread effects in your body, including acne.

Besides breakouts, other signs of estrogen dominance are: weight gain in the hips, waist and thighs, irregular or abnormal menstrual periods, breast swelling or tenderness, fibrocystic breasts, PMS, mood swings, bloating and fatigue.

Causes of estrogen dominance

- Exposure to environmental toxins that mimic estrogen, such as xenoestrogens
- Eating conventional meat and dairy products

- Taking hormonal birth control pills
- Drinking too much alcohol
- Excess body fat
- Gene mutations such as COMT and MTHFR
- Chronic stress (your body uses progesterone to make the stress hormone cortisol, which causes low progesterone and estrogen dominance)

HORMONE IMBALANCE 2: ANDROGEN EXCESS

Androgens are referred to as "male sex hormones", but in reality both men and women have them in their bodies. One condition associated with excess androgens is polycystic ovarian syndrome, or PCOS.

PCOS is the most common hormone disorder in women of childbearing age and is the leading cause of female infertility in the United States. While the exact cause is unknown, several factors, including genetics, diet, stress and environmental toxins, may be involved.

A majority of women with PCOS have insulin resistance. This makes the ovaries secrete too much testosterone, an androgen hormone, and can also inhibit the production of sex hormone binding globulin (SHBG), which acts as a mop for hormones like testosterone. Without enough SHBG, testosterone levels increase, causing acne and other symptoms associated with high testosterone.

Signs and symptoms of PCOS

- Infrequent, irregular or prolonged menstrual cycle

- Signs of excess androgens: excess facial or body hair (hirsutism), male-pattern baldness, acne
- Polycystic ovaries seen on ultrasound

SUMMARY

The root causes of acne are modifiable with diet, supplements and lifestyle interventions.

Key takeaways

- Acne is a symptom of an underlying imbalance in your gut, immune system, hormone system or mind-body connection
- The root causes of acne are inflammation, oxidative stress and hormone imbalance

CHAPTER 3

THE CLEAR SKIN PROTOCOL

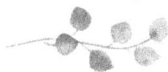

The Clear Skin Protocol is an intensive 4-week program to reset your skin.

It takes about this amount of time for your skin to undergo a full renewal cycle, so following the protocol for the entire duration is key. For severe cases of acne, consider continuing the protocol for longer (8 weeks).

The protocol is based on five interventions:

- Gut Repair
- Therapeutic Diet
- Supplements
- Topical Treatments
- Lifestyle Hacks

For the fastest results, implement all of the interventions at once.

Here's how it works:

- **For gut repair,** you'll assess what gut imbalance you have. This dictates which of the three food and supplement plans you'll follow.
- **For therapeutic diet,** you'll follow a specific food plan to heal your gut.
- **For supplements,** you'll follow a supplement plan to support digestion, correct any nutrient deficiencies and treat your gut imbalance.
- **For topical treatments,** you'll simplify your skincare routine and use natural skincare therapies to repair your skin from the outside.
- **For lifestyle hacks,** you'll learn how to make informed choices that support your skin and overall health.

This may feel overwhelming (and I know how you feel).

When I was 22, I decided to try the ketogenic diet. I had a tight budget and zero meal planning or cooking experience. I walked into the grocery store with a list of foods to shop for and I had to read nutrition labels for the first time in my life. I quickly realized that half of the items I was used to buying were not allowed. It took me two hours to finish shopping, but it was much faster after that first trip.

I also had to learn how to cook. Until then, my go-to recipe was nachos. I cooked some really bad meals (to this day I can't stand meatloaf), but over time I found recipes that I could cook, mostly simple dishes like scrambled eggs, stews and soups.

My point is: *I've been there, and I know how much work goes into something like this.*

Don't beat yourself up if you don't follow things 100%—mistakes are okay! It's not the end of the world if you don't buy organic, can't afford all of the supplements or pull an all-nighter.

Instead, focus on the changes that you *can* make, like eating more real foods, drinking more water, choosing skincare products with clean ingredients and practicing meditation every day to manage stress.

Whatever the case, **doing something is better than doing nothing.** Do what works best for your budget, time and lifestyle. If you can't do all of the interventions at once, start by doing one. Then, add the rest in as you're able.

Now that you've gotten an overview of the protocol, it's important to make sure that you're prepared beforehand. In the next chapter, you'll learn how to set yourself up for success.

SUMMARY

The Clear Skin Protocol is an intensive 4-week program to reset your skin. It involves major changes to your diet and lifestyle.

Key takeaways

- The five interventions of the protocol are gut repair, therapeutic diet, supplements, topical treatments and lifestyle hacks
- Choose to do one, some, or all of the interventions depending on what works best for your budget, time and lifestyle—the more you do, the faster your results

CHAPTER 4

BEFORE YOU GET STARTED

"By failing to prepare, you are preparing to fail."

BENJAMIN FRANKLIN

Give yourself at least a week or two to prepare before starting the protocol. Figure out as many details beforehand as you can.

CHOOSE A START DATE

Start the protocol during a time that you won't be doing anything out of the ordinary, like traveling, preparing for finals or finishing a major project at work. Mark the day on your calendar so that you have time to mentally prepare.

PRINT OUT YOUR FOOD PLAN

Printable versions of the food plans are available on my website, renellestayton.com. Tape them to your fridge for easy reference.

LEARN HOW TO READ NUTRITION LABELS

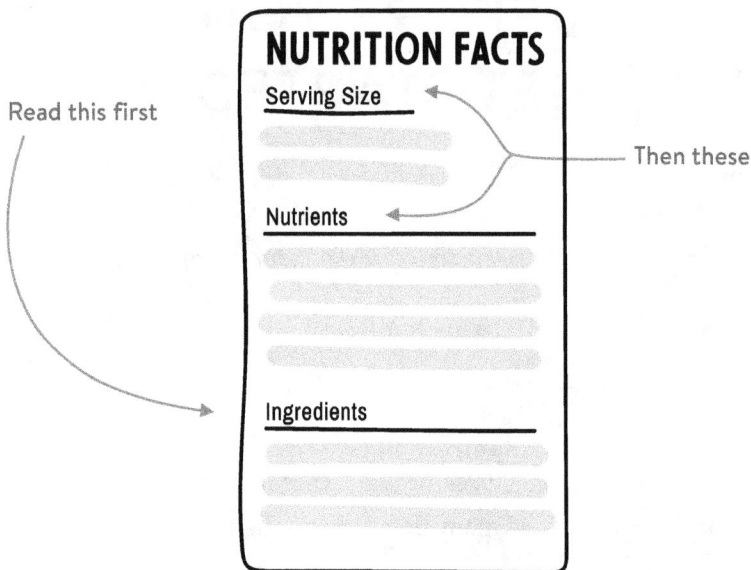

Read this first

NUTRITION FACTS

Serving Size

Then these

Nutrients

Ingredients

First, look at the ingredients on the bottom. The first ingredients listed are what there is the greatest amount of, followed in descending order by those present in smaller amounts. For example, if you're eating a protein bar and the first ingredient is almond butter, then it's mostly made out of almond butter. **The ingredient list is the most important part because it tells you exactly what the food is made out of—it will be your first tip-off if you should include or avoid something.** You will see if there are healthy ingredients, unhealthy ingredients, or any hidden sources of foods not allowed on your food plan (such as sugar, dairy, gluten).

Next, look at the serving size at the top. Serving size is key! It tells you how much of the food constitutes one serving. For example, it might say "per 10 crackers" or "per 2 tablespoons."

Last, look at the nutrients in the middle. You'll see how much protein, fat, carbohydrates, fiber, vitamins and minerals are in **one serving.** Also included is the amount of sugar and *added sugar,* which is exactly what it sounds like: sugar that's been added.

KITCHEN GEAR

I recommend having a high-speed blender. A pressure cooker is nice to have but not mandatory.

MEAL PREP

Choose one day per week to be your meal prep day. Sunday is a good day to do this. Use the meal plans and recipes provided, or look up recipes on your own. Make big enough batches of the meal prep items to last the entire week, such as:

- Gluten-free grains - oatmeal, rice, *quinoa
- Roasted vegetables - broccoli, *butternut squash, *sweet potatoes
- Salad dressings - *mustard vinaigrette
- Sauces - *artichoke dip, *pesto
- *Bone broth

- *Mediterranean chicken sausage
- *Sweet potato latkes

  *Recipe included

KEEP IT SIMPLE

You don't need to make new recipes every day. Choose three to four dinner recipes and that will give you enough leftovers to last the week.

Easy meals

- Breakfast - protein shake
- Lunch - leftovers from dinner on top of a big salad
- Snack - nuts
- Dinner - one-pot meal like stew or leftovers

Simple Snacks

- Nuts
- Unsweetened coconut yogurt with berries
- Rolled up turkey slices dipped in mustard
- Cinnamon rice cakes with almond butter
- Carrots and hummus
- Hard-boiled eggs with salt and pepper

IDENTIFY YOUR EATING TRIGGERS

Do you tend to binge late at night? Or is it during the afternoon slump at work?

Figure out what situations make it the hardest for you to make healthy choices. Make an action plan for what you'll do during those times. If you know that you crave sweets around 3pm, eat a snack at 2pm.

ORDER SUPPLEMENTS

If you're ordering supplements, have them shipped to you before you start the protocol. If you're buying them in person, see if your local grocery store or health food store stocks what you need.

PATCH TEST NEW SKINCARE PRODUCTS

Review the list of topical treatments you'll use during the protocol (see Chapter 8). Patch test anything new before using it on your entire face, such as a new cleanser, rosehip seed oil, honey or niacinamide, to name a few. I recommend doing this at least one week before starting the protocol.

- Apply the new product to a small area on either your cheek or chin (areas that are most prone to breakouts because there's a higher concentration of oil-producing glands).

- Continue to apply it as often as you would during the protocol in the same area to see how your skin reacts. Breakouts from new products will usually occur within this time period. Immediately stop using the product if it causes any type of reaction, breakouts or otherwise.

- If your skin doesn't react after one week, then it's okay to use it on your entire face.

WHAT TO EXPECT

- **Week 1** your motivation is highest. This works in your favor because the learning curve is the steepest. You're learning how to grocery shop for a food plan, meal plan, and cook new recipes (maybe for the first time ever!). You're also adding in supplements and changing up your normal skincare routine. While these changes may be fun for some, for others it can feel like an uphill battle. You've got this!

- **Week 2** can be tough, especially if you are experiencing brain fog, headache, irritability, gas, bloating, body aches or fatigue. This can happen when your body detoxifies, especially as Candida or SIBO die-off. The dying yeast and bacteria can produce toxins at a rate too fast for your body to process and eliminate. While mildly unpleasant, these symptoms are a good sign because it means that the unwanted yeast and bacteria are getting eradicated. However, not everyone will experience this. You may feel great!

- **Week 3** you'll have settled into a familiar routine and the protocol is starting to feel like second nature. You may notice that you don't have any new breakouts and that old breakouts are healing faster.

- **Week 4** your skin is clearer than it has ever been before! An added bonus is that your body also feels better than ever.

- **Week 5** you'll start to reintroduce the eliminated foods. This is where the real detective work comes into play. You'll learn what foods work for your skin and body (and what doesn't) so you can personalize your diet that you'll follow after the protocol to maintain clear skin.

Reduce Detox Symptoms

Take Epsom salt baths, move regularly, sleep at least eight hours every night and supplement with activated charcoal (1000 mg daily for detox purposes). Take activated charcoal at least two hours away from medications and other supplements, as it can interfere with their effectiveness. It can turn your poop black (so don't be alarmed) and can be constipating, so drink lots of water.

TRACK YOUR PROGRESS

Take "before" and "after" pictures. Include all areas on your face and body that have acne. Make sure to take the pictures in the same place with the same lighting so that you have an accurate comparison. If you want to, share them with me on my website. I love seeing your progress pictures!

SUMMARY

Preparation will set you up for success. Changing the way that you eat is often the biggest challenge, so familiarize yourself with your food plan ahead of time.

Key takeaways

- Learn how to read nutrition labels
- Review the list of topical treatments you'll use during the protocol (see Chapter 8) and patch test anything new before using it on your entire face
- Track progress with "before" and "after" pictures

CHAPTER 5

GUT REPAIR

"All disease begins in the gut."

HIPPOCRATES

The first step to healing your skin is healing your gut.
Functional medicine uses the 5R framework to do this.

5R Framework for Gut Healing

- **Remove** things that negatively impact your gut environment, like food sensitivities, bacterial overgrowth or yeast

- **Replace** digestive secretions with digestive enzymes and betaine HCL

- **Reinoculate** your gut with beneficial bacteria, using probiotics and fermented foods

- **Repair** the gut barrier with things like L-glutamine, bone broth

- **Rebalance** other aspects of your life to improve gut health, such as managing stress

These are guiding principles that have already been incorporated into the Clear Skin Protocol so you don't need to remember all of this information—it's just to give you a better understanding of the "why" behind the interventions.

GUT ISSUES ASSOCIATED WITH ACNE

- Leaky gut
- Candida overgrowth
- Small intestinal bacterial overgrowth (SIBO)

Leaky Gut

You'll follow the leaky gut treatment plan *unless* you identify that you're dealing with Candida or SIBO, which can complicate leaky gut. If this is the case, follow their treatment plans instead. If you're unsure of what to do, follow the leaky gut plan.

While there are lab tests that help identify gut issues, like comprehensive stool testing, these tests are expensive and often require a healthcare professional who can order the testing and interpret your results. An elimination diet, which is the leaky gut food plan, is absolutely free and will give you even more detailed and accurate advice about your diet, skin and overall health.

The elimination diet allows you to identify what works best for your biochemistry. By removing foods that are the most common food sensitivities, you give your gut a chance to repair itself.

You add these foods back in later to see if they cause any type of reaction, so you can personalize your diet to keep your skin clear for the long-term.

For example, when I did the elimination diet, I learned that I was sensitive to dairy and eggs. I tried adding them back again after waiting several weeks, but they still made me break out and gave me brain fog. I still don't include them in my diet.

Lab Tests for Leaky Gut

- **Comprehensive stool testing.** This is the laboratory gold standard for identifying gut imbalances and infections. Unlike stool tests ordered in the conventional setting, it looks at different biomarkers in your stool to determine the amounts of commensal bacteria present, if there is an imbalance between the good and bad microbes in your gut (also called dysbiosis), how well you digest and absorb food, and if there is inflammation present. This test must be ordered and interpreted by a qualified healthcare provider. I recommend the Comprehensive Stool Analysis by Doctor's Data or GI-MAP by Diagnostic Solutions.

- **Lactulose-mannitol testing.** This urine test measures the ability of non-metabolized sugar molecules to permeate the gut barrier.

- **Blood test for zonulin and lipopolysaccharides (LPS).** Both will be elevated if leaky gut is present. Elevated zonulin causes the tight junctions

Continued on following page

in between your gut barrier cells to break apart, causing leaky gut. LPS is released by gut bacteria and will be detectable in the bloodstream if there is a breech in the gut barrier.

- **IgG food sensitivity testing.** This test helps identify which foods you're sensitive to by testing your blood. Many sensitivities to different foods can indicate that leaky gut is an issue. You can order this test for yourself online, such as the Food Sensitivity Test by EverlyWell.

LEAKY GUT TREATMENT PLAN

- **Follow the Leaky Gut Food Plan outlined in Chapter 6.1.**
- **Follow the Leaky Gut Supplement Plan outlined in Chapter 7.**
- **Don't take antibiotics, birth control pills or NSAIDs unless medically necessary.** These drugs can harm your gut. Antibiotics disrupt your microbiome and increase your risk of developing Candida and SIBO. Birth control pills can contain estrogen which doubles the risk of developing Candida overgrowth. Even at low doses, NSAIDs like ibuprofen can cause bleeding and ulcers.
- **Don't eat too many raw vegetables.** Raw vegetables are difficult for an inflamed leaky gut to digest. They can cause bloating, gas and abdominal discom-

fort. Try to cook vegetables beforehand so that your gut has an easier time breaking them down.

- **Drink bone broth every day.** Bone broth is rich in collagen, gelatin and fat-soluble vitamins that restore your gut barrier.

- **Try intermittent fasting.** It gives your gut a break from digesting, which speeds recovery of the gut barrier. Start by fasting for 12 hours and eating within the remaining 12 hour window. For example, eat from 7am-7pm and fast from 7pm-7am. You can drink water during the fasting period.

- **Create space for quiet reflection and rest.** Unmanaged stress derails any gut-healing protocol and increases the likelihood of developing leaky gut. Set aside time every day to meditate, practice yoga, take an Epsom salt bath or play music—whatever works best for you.

SPECIAL CONSIDERATIONS: CANDIDA AND SIBO

Candida

Candida is a type of yeast that is present in your microbiome in small amounts. Normally, it stays in balance with the other microbes in your gut, like bacteria, and helps your body break down food and absorb nutrients.

The problem is when there is too much Candida. It can overpower the good bacteria in your gut, leading to leaky gut and other problems. Causes of Candida overgrowth include: eating a high sugar and processed diet, use of medications like antibiotics, birth control pills or steroids, and stress.

First, consider if any of the following apply to your medical history:

- Use of antibiotics for acne for one month or longer
- Use of broad-spectrum antibiotics for respiratory or urinary tract infections (for two months or longer or four courses in one year)
- Use of birth control pills for more than six months
- Use of corticosteroids (like prednisone or decadron) for more than two weeks
- Chronic vaginal yeast infections or vaginal itching
- Chronic fungal infections (like athlete's foot, ringworm or nail fungal infections)

Next, evaluate if you are experiencing symptoms related to Candida. Unfortunately many of the major symptoms are nonspecific and overlap with a number of other conditions that aren't Candida. To help you weed out if Candida is the problem, determine if you experience these symptoms on a *regular* basis and if your medical history puts you at risk. If yes to both, there is a good chance that Candida is the culprit.

SYMPTOMS OF CANDIDA

- Strong cravings for sugar, refined carbohydrates, alcohol

- Brain fog, trouble concentrating or focusing, poor memory
- Fatigue
- Depression and/or anxiety
- Dizziness or light-headedness
- Sinus pressure or congestion
- Frequent sore throat
- Muscle pain or weakness
- Vaginal itching or burning
- Low libido

Symptoms are provoked or worsened if you are exposed to perfumes or chemical odors, or if you are in a damp or moldy environment.

Lab Tests for Candida

- **Comprehensive stool testing.** This is the most accurate way to diagnose Candida.
- **Blood test for Candida antibodies (IgA, IgG, IgM).**
- **Complete blood count.** Certain findings, like low lymphocytes and high neutrophils, can indicate Candida.

If you determine Candida is the problem, you'll follow the Candida treatment plan below. The goal of treatment is 1) to get rid of the overgrowth by following an anti-Candida diet and taking natural antifungals and 2) restoring balance to the microbiome.

CANDIDA TREATMENT PLAN

- **Follow the Candida Food Plan outlined in Chapter 6.2.**

- **Follow the Candida Supplement Plan outlined in Chapter 7.**

- **Don't take antibiotics, birth control pills or NSAIDs unless medically necessary.** Antibiotics disrupt your microbiome and increase your risk of developing Candida. Birth control pills can contain estrogen which doubles your risk of developing Candida.

- **Get rid of the Candida overgrowth.** Caprylic acid is a natural antifungal used to get rid of Candida. It is a medium-chain fatty acid found in coconut and palm oils that destroys yeast cell walls.

- **Prevent recurrence.** Recurrence is common, so continuing to limit sugar, refined carbohydrates and certain kinds of alcohol (like wine) after the protocol may be in order. For severe or recurrent cases of Candida that are not responsive to natural antifungals and the anti-Candida diet, you may need to consider prescription antifungals.

- **Create space for quiet reflection and rest.** Finding a way to manage stress is essential for gut, skin and hormonal health. Do what works best for you.

Small intestinal bacterial overgrowth

Small intestinal bacterial overgrowth (SIBO) is a common gut imbalance that occurs when bacteria overgrow and cause problems in your small intestine. These bacteria have usually migrated up from the large intestine. The bacteria release endotoxins that cause your gut to become leaky and inflamed. This impairs nutrient absorption and makes foods that are normally considered healthy (like garlic, broccoli and avocados) problematic. The bacteria ferment sugar and starches in these foods, which produces hydrogen and methane gas. This is what causes the trademark symptoms of SIBO: gas and bloating.

Causes of SIBO include low stomach acid, decreased bile flow and a deficiency in the migrating motor complex (MMC) in your gut. The MMC is what moves food and other waste products from your small intestine to your large intestine between meals. MMC stagnation creates the perfect environment for bacterial overgrowth.

Consider if any of the following apply to your medical history:

- History of irritable bowel syndrome (IBS)
- History of a gastrointestinal infection like traveler's diarrhea, food poisoning or the stomach flu (viral gastroenteritis)

Next, evaluate if you have any symptoms of SIBO.

- Frequent gas and bloating, especially after eating sugar and starches (including grains, bread, pasta, desserts, sugar alcohols like xylitol or sorbitol, fiber supplements)
- Chronic constipation and/or diarrhea
- Digestive symptoms improve when you take antibiotics
- Blood work has shown chronically low levels of B12, iron or ferritin

Lab Tests for SIBO

- **Lactulose breath test.** This test measures whether hydrogen or methane gas is produced by SIBO as they ferment sugar and starches. You fast beforehand and then breathe into a test tube to determine your baseline levels. Then, you drink a sugar solution which feeds the SIBO. You repeat breath samples over a period of several hours to see if the levels of hydrogen or methane gas increase.
- **Comprehensive stool test.** Elevated levels of good bacteria can sometimes indicate SIBO.

If your medical history and symptoms indicate that SIBO is the problem, you'll follow the SIBO treatment plan below. The goals of treatment are 1) to get rid of the bacterial overgrowth by following a low-FODMAP diet and taking herbal antibiotics, 2) healing the gut barrier, and 3) restoring normal function of the MMC.

SIBO TREATMENT PLAN

- **Follow the SIBO Food Plan outlined in Chapter 6.3.**

- **Follow the SIBO Supplement Plan outlined in Chapter 7.** With SIBO, it's especially important to test yourself for low stomach acid using the baking soda test or the betaine HCL test (outlined in Chapter 7), since low stomach acid is an underlying cause of SIBO.

- **Don't take antibiotics, acid-blockers, birth control pills or NSAIDs unless medically necessary.** However, for recurrent or severe cases of SIBO that are not responsive to a low-FODMAP diet and herbal antibiotics, prescription antibiotics may be indicated. Acid blockers increase your risk of developing SIBO because stomach acid prevents bacterial overgrowth in your small intestine.

- **Get rid of bad bacteria.** Herbal antibiotic blends containing things like berberine, oregano oil and wormwood help "weed out" the bacterial overgrowth. They are a gentler and natural alternative to antibiotics. You'll learn about how to take these in Chapter 7. When compared to the antibiotic rifaximin, herbal antibiotic therapy has been found to be as effective at treating SIBO [1]. For severe or recurrent cases of SIBO, you may have to consider antibiotics. Rifaximin and/or neomycin are the primary antibiotics prescribed to treat SIBO, depending on the type of SIBO you have (hydrogen vs. methane predominant). Unlike most antibiotics, rifaximin is non-absorbed and narrow-spectrum, so it won't cause as much harm to your gut as a broad-spectrum antibiotic would.

- **Restore normal function of the migrating motor complex (MMC).** To support MMC function, practice mindful eating and careful chewing, along with exercises that stimulate the vagus nerve, like singing and gargling [2,3]. The MMC only works when you're in a fasted state, so space meals at least 4-5 hours apart and fast for 12 hours overnight. Promotility agents (also known as prokinetics) can be used after treatment with herbal or prescription antibiotics to prevent recurrence of SIBO by stimulating the cleansing waves of the MMC. Natural prokinetics include ginger, Swedish bitters, bitter greens and fennel seeds.

- **Create space for quiet reflection and rest.** Finding a way to manage stress is essential for gut, skin and hormonal health. Do what works best for you.

SUPPORT PATHWAYS OF ELIMINATION

Regular poops

Pooping every day is an important part of maintaining gut health. You should poop 1-2 times daily. If you poop less often, this allows waste products (like excess hormones and toxins) to get reabsorbed in your gut, which contributes to acne.

To improve pooping regularity, eat more fiber-containing foods, drink enough water and exercise regularly.

WHAT IS FIBER?

Fiber is a type of carbohydrate found in most plant foods. Many people are deficient in fiber, getting only about 15 grams daily. Aim for 30-50 grams daily, working your way up slowly to this amount.

For leaky gut, focus on eating more soluble fiber foods rather than insoluble fiber foods, which can be difficult for a leaky gut to digest.

For SIBO, you may be limiting certain fiber-containing foods as you follow the low-FODMAP diet. Focus on including fiber-containing foods that you can have, and avoid fiber supplements that contain inulin or fructooligosaccharides (FOS)/galactooligosaccharides (GOS).

Constipation

For constipation, take 200mg of magnesium citrate once before bed. Increase the dose slowly until you have a soft stool, up to 600mg max. If you take too much, you can get diarrhea, so back off the dose if this happens. Most people are deficient in magnesium as it is, even if you eat lots of magnesium-rich foods. If you've tried different things for constipation without success, consider having your thyroid levels checked.

Drink more water

To calculate your daily water requirement, divide your weight (in pounds) in half and drink that many ounces of water per day. For example, a 160 lb person should drink 80 oz of water daily, or 10 cups (8 oz = 1 cup).

Next time you go pee, look at the color of your urine to see if you're hydrated enough. Urine should be clear to light yellow; dark colored urine indicates that you need to drink more water.

If you can, invest in a water filter that you can afford. There are less expensive options, like a charcoal filter, and more expensive options, like a reverse osmosis filter. Look for filtration systems that are National Science Foundation (NSF) certified, whose standards establish minimum requirements for contaminant filtration. I use an NSF-certified countertop filter by ZeroWater.

What About Tap and Bottled Water?

Tap water can contain pesticides, prescription drugs and heavy metals that cause hormone imbalance and toxin overload. These contaminants often have no legal limits and their long-term health effects are not known. You can refer to the Environmental Working Group (EWG) Tap Water Database (ewg.org/tapwater) to see what's in your city's tap water.

Bottled water can contain bisphenol A (BPA), which mimics estrogen. In fact, BPA was used as a synthetic form of estrogen in the 1930s. BPA is also found in plastic food containers, canned goods and receipt paper. Use glass or stainless steel water bottles and food containers instead of plastic and avoid reheating or storing food in plastic.

SUMMARY

Follow the leaky gut food and supplement plan unless you determine that Candida or SIBO are an issue. If that is the case, follow those plans instead. Regular poops and adequate hydration are essential for maintaining gut health.

Key takeaways

- Heal your gut to heal your skin
- Don't take antibiotics, acid-blockers, birth control pills or NSAIDs unless medically necessary
- Poop 1-2 times daily and drink more water

CHAPTER 6

THERAPEUTIC DIET

"Your fork, the most powerful tool to transform your health and change the world."

MARK HYMAN, MD

EAT REAL, WHOLE FOODS

These are foods that come in their natural, unprocessed form. Think of things like vegetables, fruits, meat, eggs, nuts and seeds. They don't come in a package with a list of ingredients that you don't recognize or can't pronounce.

BUILD YOUR CLEAR SKIN PLATE

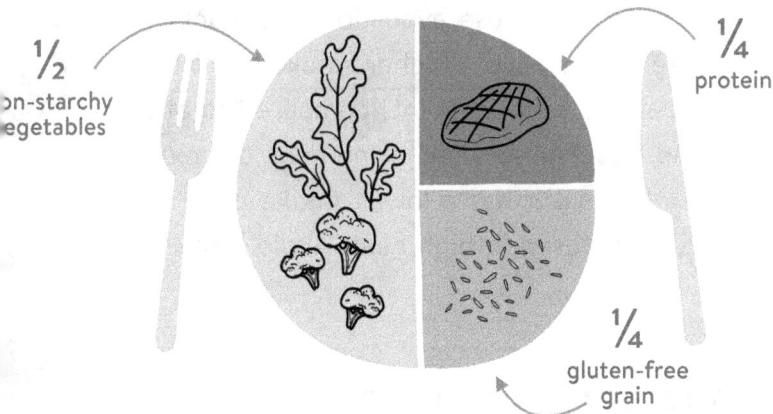

½
non-starchy vegetables

¼
protein

¼
gluten-free grain

Fill half your plate with non-starchy vegetables, one quarter with protein, one quarter with a gluten-free grain (or starchy vegetable) and add one serving of fat.

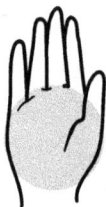

PROTEIN
portion

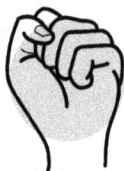

NON-STARCHY VEGETABLES
portion

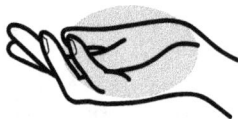

GLUTEN-FREE GRAIN or STARCHY VEGETABLE
portion

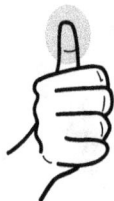

FAT
portion

Use your hand as a tool for estimating portion sizes.

Cooking Oils and Fats

Look for oils that are packaged in dark glass bottles with a tight seal. Keep oils stored in the dark, away from the stove and other hot areas.

For high heat, use avocado oil, coconut oil or ghee. These have a higher smoke point (also known as the burning point) compared to other oils and fats. For very low or no heat, use extra-virgin olive oil. It has a lower smoke point and shouldn't be used in high heat. Avoid trans fats and highly processed oils like canola, safflower, sunflower and soybean. If you do choose to use them, make sure they are certified organic and non-GMO.

CHOOSE THERAPEUTIC FOODS FOR ACNE

It's important to consider the *quality* of the foods that you eat. All food belongs to one or more of the following macronutrient groups: protein, fats and carbohydrates. Sources of protein are meat, poultry, fish, legumes and eggs. Sources of fat are avocado, oils, nuts and seeds. Sources of carbohydrates are grains, fruits, vegetables and legumes.

In addition to macronutrients, food also contains micronutrients, which are vitamins and minerals. These play an important role in maintaining your bodily functions, especially as it relates to clear skin. Micronutrients decrease inflammation and oxidative stress, promote hormonal balance and aid in skin repair. I encourage you to include micronutrient-rich, therapeutic foods for acne in your diet as often as possible.

Therapeutic foods for acne

- Liver and other organ meats
- SMASH fish (salmon, mackerel, anchovies, sardines, herring)
- Bone broth
- Different colored fruits and vegetables

- Turmeric
- Green tea

Vegetarian or Vegan?

Focus on including the therapeutic foods that aren't animal products and make modifications to the food plans and recipes as you see fit. Incorporate more protein and fats (lentils, nuts, seeds, avocados, extra virgin olive oil) and be mindful of the glycemic load of your diet, limiting gluten-free whole grains and starchy beans to keep blood sugar levels balanced.

About the therapeutic foods

LIVER AND OTHER ORGAN MEATS

Organ meats contain anywhere from 10 to 100 times more nutrients than muscle meat. Liver is one of the most nutrient-dense foods on the planet. **It's packed with skin-healing nutrients, like zinc and vitamin A, which help the skin turnover and prevent acne from developing.** People with acne have lower levels of these nutrients in their blood and skin [1-4]. I recommend eating liver at least once or twice per week.

The taste can be an acquired one, so try sautéing it in a little bit of ghee with onions and garlic (or green onions if low-FOD-MAP) and dip it in a stone-ground mustard. You can also add small pieces of liver to ground beef in pasta sauces, or blend it into a pâté.

Buying meat and organ meats from grass-fed animals is better for your health, the environment and the animals. Compared to industrially-raised "feedlot" animals who are confined indoors and fed a diet of genetically modified corn and soy, grass-fed animals are raised outdoors grazing on grass in open pastures for food. Grass-fed meat has a better fatty acid profile, more precursors for vitamins and more antioxidants compared to feedlot meat [5].

Choose grass-fed, sustainably raised meat and organ meats, eating them in moderation.

SMASH FISH

SMASH stands for salmon, mackerel, anchovies, sardines and herring. These fish are highest in omega-3s, which are anti-inflammatory and promote clear skin. Most people do not get enough omega-3s in their diet.

Choose wild-caught or sustainably raised farmed fish. Pass on "feedlot" fish which can contain high amounts of polychlorinated biphenyl (PCB), a harmful compound.

Fish that are high in mercury should be avoided, including: tilefish, king mackerel, grouper, marlin, swordfish and tuna.

For information on how to buy environmentally friendly seafood, visit the Monterey Bay Aquarium Seafood Watch site (seafoodwatch.org).

BONE BROTH

Bone broth contains minerals, amino acids and gelatin which are nourishing for an inflamed gut. It is made by simmering soup bones in water with vegetables and spices. Over time, the stock becomes infused with nutrients from the marrow, connective tissue and bones.

If you can, drink bone broth every day during the protocol. You can make your own broth at home or buy it from the grocery store. I've included my bone broth recipe in the recipe section.

DIFFERENT COLORED FRUITS AND VEGETABLES

Fresh fruits and vegetables contain phytonutrients that help heal acne. Eating a variety of colors ("eating the rainbow") and choosing deeply pigmented produce ensures that you get the widest range of phytonutrients in your diet and the most health benefits.

- For acne, eat more dark purple, dark green, red and yellow foods
- For gut health, eat more red, white and brown foods

Eat the Rainbow

- Purple: beets, berries, figs, plums
- Green: artichokes, avocados, broccoli, cucumbers, dark leafy greens, limes, zucchinis
- Red: apples, cherries, pomegranate seeds, raspberries, strawberries
- Yellow: bananas, lemons, pineapples, squashes
- White: beans, cauliflower, coconut, garlic, mushrooms, onions
- Brown: ginger root, nuts, pears, seeds, tahini, gluten-free whole grains

When you can, buy organic. Organic means that the produce is grown without the use of genetically modified seeds, synthetic chemicals (like pesticides) or growth regulators. Studies have shown that people who eat organic, compared to conventional, have 6-9 times less pesticide metabolites in their urine [6-8].

Glyphosate is one pesticide that you should avoid at all costs. It's the active ingredient in the weed-killing product, Roundup, which is routinely sprayed on conventional crops like corn, soy and wheat. High levels of glyphosate have been correlated with birth defects, cancer and fertility problems [9-12].

Use the Environmental Working Group (EWG) Clean Fifteen and Dirty Dozen list to help you decide what produce is okay to buy conventionally grown and what you should buy organic. This list is updated every year.

−EWG SHOPPER'S GUIDE−

CLEAN FIFTEEN	
(lowest in pesticides, okay to buy conventionally grown)	
1. Avocados	9. Cauliflower
2. Sweet corn	10. Cantaloupe
3. Pineapples	11. Broccoli
4. Onions	12. Mushrooms
5. Papaya	13. Cabbage
6. Sweet peas (frozen)	14. Honeydew melon
7. Eggplant	15. Kiwi
8. Asparagus	

DIRTY DOZEN	
(highest in pesticides, buy organic)	
1. Strawberries	7. Peaches
2. Spinach	8. Cherries
3. Kale	9. Pears
4. Nectarines	10. Tomatoes
5. Apples	11. Celery
6. Grapes	12. Potatoes

Money-saving tips for buying organic

- Buy pantry staples in bulk. These include gluten-free whole grains, extra-virgin olive oil, coconut oil, frozen berries, protein powder and bone broth.

- Stock up during sales and freeze whatever you don't use.

- Get frozen instead of fresh produce. Frozen produce retains its nutrient value because it's frozen at peak ripeness.

TURMERIC

Turmeric has been used medicinally and as a culinary spice in Asia and parts of the Middle East for nearly 4,000 years. Traditional Chinese and Ayurvedic medicines have used it as an anti-inflammatory for skin and joint disorders, as well as an analgesic and digestive aid.

Curcuminoids, a bioactive component of turmeric, inhibit the nuclear factor kappa B (NF-kB) pathway, which is responsible for the inflammatory response [13]. Add turmeric to your cooking as much as possible to get the anti-inflammatory benefits. You can try the golden milk in the recipe section.

GREEN TEA

Green tea is rich in polyphenols that have anti-inflammatory, antioxidant and antimicrobial effects on the skin [14-16]. The most abundant of these polyphenols is epigallocatechin gallate (EGCG). Studies have found that EGCG inhibits growth of bacteria involved in acne, decreases sebum production and reduces inflammation [17,18].

Matcha is a type of green tea that contains 100 times more EGCG than regular green tea [19]. Add 1 tsp of matcha powder to a cup of hot (but not boiling) water and blend with a handheld frother or bamboo whisk. For a creamier version of this drink, see the matcha latte in the recipe section.

HONORABLE MENTIONS

Eggs and fermented foods are also important for skin and gut health. However, the leaky gut plan eliminates eggs and the Candida plan eliminates most fermented foods. If your plan allows them, include them in your diet.

EGGS

Eggs are one of the best sources of protein. Yolks contain important skin-healing nutrients, like omega-3s, fat-soluble vitamins, minerals and antioxidants, so make sure to eat them! Keep the yolks runny to retain the most nutrients. I recommend using eggs that are labeled pasture-raised and certified humane, which is different from cage-free and free-range.

Pasture-raised, certified humane indicates that the chickens were free to roam and feed outside on open fields (they're allocated 108 square feet per bird). Pastured eggs contain double the amount of omega-3s and higher amounts of vitamins A and E (both important for skin health) compared to conventional eggs [20].

Cage-free only means that the chickens were not living in a cage, it doesn't specify how much space they actually have or if they can go outside.

Free-range means that chickens were given access to outdoors (which may just be a cemented area) but it doesn't guarantee that the chicken ever stepped outside.

FERMENTED FOODS

Fermented foods are a staple in traditional diets around the world. They're filled with beneficial bacteria that nourish your gut microbiome. Examples of fermented foods include: sauerkraut, kimchi, miso, pickles, yogurt and kefir.

If allowed on your food plan, incorporate fermented foods into your meals every day. This can be as simple as adding a spoonful of sauerkraut to any meal or having a bowl of coconut yogurt as a snack.

ELIMINATE PROBLEMATIC FOODS

Now that you know what foods to include, let's talk about what foods to avoid.

Dairy, sugar, gluten and alcohol are problematic for your gut and skin, so you won't find them in any of the food plans. Depending on what food plan you're following, you'll also be eliminating other foods for the four weeks.

Why no dairy, sugar, gluten and alcohol?

As you already learned in Chapter 2, these things make acne worse. Let's briefly review why you'll avoid them during the protocol.

DAIRY

Dairy contains too many hormones, inflammatory proteins (casein and whey) and growth factors that worsen acne. It also raises insulin levels as much as high-sugar foods do, which triggers a hormonal cascade that causes acne.

The only exception to the no-dairy rule is ghee. Ghee is clarified butter that's had the water and milk solids removed from it. It doesn't have the inflammatory casein and whey proteins that normal butter does, so ghee is generally well tolerated. It does depend on the person, so see if it works for you. You can make your own ghee at home or buy it at the grocery store. Use grass-fed butter if you make your own.

SUGAR

Eating too much sugar increases blood sugar and insulin levels too much, which causes acne.

During the protocol you're going to avoid artificial and natural sugars. There are the obvious forms of sugar, like cookies, cake and candy, and less obvious forms, like white bread, fruit juice and commercial salad dressings. Remember to read ingredient labels to see the total sugar amount and added sugar amount. A general rule of thumb is: if it tastes sweet, avoid it. Use your common sense here.

Other words for "sugar":

- Agave
- Brown sugar
- Cane sugar, dehydrated cane juice
- Corn syrup, high fructose corn syrup
- Date sugar
- Fruit juice, fruit juice concentrate
- Honey
- Malt
- Molasses
- Things that end in "-ose", like dextrose, fructose, glucose, maltose, sucrose
- Syrup
- Turbinado

Refined Flour

Refined flour (like white flour) acts like sugar inside of the body. It's stripped of most of the bran and germ which contains nutrients and fiber. Fiber is important because it slows down the release of sugar into the bloodstream. It's best to avoid anything labeled "refined", which means that the product has undergone this stripping process. Choose whole grain flours instead.

Stevia is the only sweetener allowed during the protocol. It doesn't spike blood sugar and is minimally absorbed. It comes in liquid, powdered or whole leaf form. Use liquid stevia for beverages and powdered stevia for baking. Whole leaf is harder to find but can be ordered online. Some stevia brands contain fillers like erythritol, which is problematic for people with SIBO, so read ingredient labels.

A little goes a long way, so use stevia **in moderation.** Use up to 10 drops of liquid stevia or 1 packet of powdered stevia per day (equivalent to about 2 tsp of sugar).

How to Beat Sugar Cravings

- Eat more sour foods like lemons and limes
- Eat more protein-rich foods like meat, fish and legumes
- Focus on fiber rich foods like ground flaxseed, wild rice and sweet potatoes
- Eat a serving of healthy fat with every meal (such as 1 T of extra virgin olive oil or 1/2 an avocado)
- Add cinnamon to food, which stabilizes blood sugar

GLUTEN

Gluten increases the release of a protein called zonulin [21,22]. Zonulin opens the tight junctions in the gut lining, allowing foreign substances to pass through into the bloodstream and activate the immune system. This condition is also known as leaky gut.

GLUTEN-CONTAINING GRAINS	GLUTEN-FREE GRAINS
Barley	Amaranth
Bulgar	Buckwheat
Durum	Oats (only if labeled gluten-free)
Kamut	
Farro	Millet
Rye	Quinoa
Spelt	Rice
Semolina	Sorghum
Wheat	Teff

Even if something is labeled gluten-free, it doesn't always mean that it's healthy. There are plenty of gluten-free junk foods and companies will often add more sugar and fat to replace gluten.

Hidden sources of gluten

- Bouillon cubes
- Cereal
- Cornbread
- Gravy
- Hot dogs
- Lunch meat
- Milk shakes

- Soup

- Soy sauce

ALCOHOL

Alcohol causes leaky gut and overburdens your liver, impacting your ability to detoxify. It also encourages bad bacteria to thrive and impairs absorption of important vitamins and minerals. Many other parts of your body are also negatively affected by drinking—like your heart, brain, pancreas and immune system, to name a few—so it's best to avoid alcohol as you're healing your gut and skin.

GO TO YOUR THERAPEUTIC FOOD PLAN

Now that you've learned about the nutrition basics, go to your specific food plan.

Chapter 6.1: Leaky Gut Food Plan
Chapter 6.2: Candida Food Plan
Chapter 6.3: SIBO Food Plan

SUMMARY

Eat real, whole foods. Use the Clear Skin Plate as a meal template and your hand as a portion guide.

Key takeaways

- Therapeutic foods for acne: liver and other organ meats, SMASH fish (salmon, mackerel, anchovies, sardines and herring), bone broth, different colored fruits and vegetables, turmeric, green tea (especially matcha)

- Use the EWG Clean Fifteen, Dirty Dozen shopping guide to help you figure out what produce is okay to buy conventionally grown and what you should buy organic

- None of the therapeutic food plans include dairy, sugar, gluten or alcohol

CHAPTER 6.1

LEAKY GUT FOOD PLAN

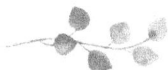

The leaky gut food plan is an elimination diet that removes the most common food sensitivities in order to repair your gut. The most common food sensitivities are dairy, gluten, eggs, corn, soy and peanuts. You'll also eliminate the foods that don't belong in any skin or gut-healing diet, like sugar and alcohol.

One way to speed healing of leaky gut is to intermittent fast. Fasting gives your gut a break from digesting so that it can repair itself. I recommend eating within a 12 hour window during the day and fasting for 12 hours overnight. For example, eat between 7am to 7pm and fast from 7pm to 7am.

Healing Foods for Leaky Gut

- Bone broth
- Ghee
- Aloe vera gel
- Lightly cooked vegetables, not raw

Continued on following page

- Probiotic-rich foods (sauerkraut, coconut yogurt)
- Prebiotic-rich foods (green bananas, cooked and cooled rice, potatoes)

* Probiotic and prebiotic-rich foods can cause gas and bloating if SIBO is present

Follow this plan for four weeks. The fifth week, you'll begin the reintroduction phase, which is detailed in Chapter 6.4.

Familiarize yourself with the grocery lists and sample meal plan included in this chapter. Printable versions are available on my website, renellestayton.com.

EAT	ELIMINATE
Grass-fed meats	All forms of sugar, natural and artificial
Fish and other seafood	
Natural fats	White flour products
Fruits	Dairy
Vegetables	Gluten
Gluten-free whole grains	Eggs
Nuts and seeds	Corn
Legumes (beans, peas, lentils)	Soy
All herbs and spices	Peanuts
Stevia	Alcohol

3-DAY MEAL PLAN

All recipes are listed in the recipe section

	DAY 1	DAY 2	DAY 3
BREAKFAST	Mediterranean Chicken Sausage with Artichoke Dip	AB&J Smoothie	Mediterranean Chicken Sausage with Artichoke Dip
LUNCH	Coconut Curry Soup	Mustard Salmon with Sweet Potato Latkes	Coconut Curry Soup
DINNER	Mustard Salmon with Sweet Potato Latkes	Coconut Curry Soup	Thai Meatballs with Baby Bok Choy and Rice

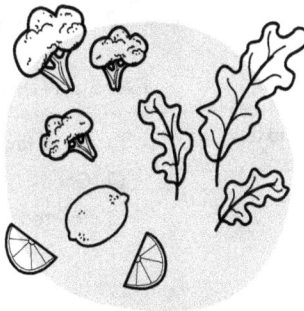

MEAL PLAN GROCERY LIST

VEGETABLES

Non-Starchy

- ☐ Baby bok choy, 6
- ☐ Carrots, 3 large
- ☐ Cilantro, 1 bunch
- ☐ Ginger root, 1 large knob
- ☐ Green onions, 2 bunches
- ☐ Parsley, 1 bunch
- ☐ Spinach, 1 bag
- ☐ Zucchini, 1

Starchy

- ☐ Acorn squash, 1
- ☐ Japanese sweet potato, 1 large
- ☐ Red potatoes, 2

FRUIT

- ☐ Bananas, 1 bunch
- ☐ Blueberries, fresh or frozen
- ☐ Limes, 1
- ☐ Lemons, 2

ANIMAL PROTEIN

- ☐ Ground beef, 1 lb
- ☐ Ground chicken thighs, 1 lb

FISH AND SEAFOOD

- ☐ Shrimp, 1 lb (peeled and deveined)

UNSWEETENED PROTEIN POWDER

- ☐ Vanilla protein powder (bone broth, hemp, pea or rice-based only)

UNSWEETENED DAIRY ALTERNATIVES

- ☐ Any (such as almond, coconut, hemp)

FISH AND SEAFOOD

- ☐ Salmon fillets, 4 (about 6 oz each)

GLUTEN-FREE GRAINS

- ☐ Arrowroot powder
- ☐ Brown rice
- ☐ Coconut flour

RAW NUTS AND SEEDS

- ☐ Almond butter
- ☐ Any nuts for snacks (except peanuts)
- ☐ Pumpkin seeds (optional)

FATS AND OILS

- ☐ Extra virgin olive oil
- ☐ Ghee
- ☐ Toasted sesame oil

HERBS, SPICES, CONDIMENTS, MISCELLANEOUS

- ☐ Artichoke hearts, 1 (14 oz) can
- ☐ Cayenne (optional)
- ☐ Coconut aminos
- ☐ Coconut milk, full fat, 1 can
- ☐ Cumin
- ☐ Dijon mustard
- ☐ Fish sauce (optional)
- ☐ Kalamata olives, pitted
- ☐ Stevia, liquid
- ☐ Tahini
- ☐ Turmeric
- ☐ Za'atar spice

FULL GROCERY LIST

VEGETABLES

Non-Starchy

- ☐ Artichoke
- ☐ Arugula
- ☐ Asparagus
- ☐ Beets
- ☐ Bell peppers
- ☐ Bok choy
- ☐ Broccoli
- ☐ Brussels sprouts
- ☐ Cabbage
- ☐ Carrots
- ☐ Cauliflower
- ☐ Celery
- ☐ Chives
- ☐ Cilantro
- ☐ Cucumber
- ☐ Dill
- ☐ Eggplant
- ☐ Fennel
- ☐ Fermented vegetables (such as sauerkraut)
- ☐ Garlic
- ☐ Green beans
- ☐ Jicama
- ☐ Kale
- ☐ Leeks
- ☐ Lettuce
- ☐ Mushrooms
- ☐ Onion
- ☐ Parsley
- ☐ Radish
- ☐ Shallots
- ☐ Spinach
- ☐ Squash (such as delicata, pumpkin, spaghetti)
- ☐ Swiss chard
- ☐ Tomato
- ☐ Zucchini

Starchy

- ☐ Acorn squash
- ☐ Butternut squash
- ☐ Parsnip
- ☐ Potatoes
- ☐ Plantain
- ☐ Yam

FRUIT

- ☐ Apples
- ☐ Apricots
- ☐ Avocado
- ☐ Banana
- ☐ Blackberries
- ☐ Blueberries
- ☐ Cantaloupe
- ☐ Cherries
- ☐ Cranberry
- ☐ Figs
- ☐ Grapefruit
- ☐ Grapes
- ☐ Kiwi
- ☐ Kumquat
- ☐ Lemons
- ☐ Limes
- ☐ Mandarin oranges
- ☐ Mango
- ☐ Melons
- ☐ Nectarines
- ☐ Oranges
- ☐ Pineapple
- ☐ Plums
- ☐ Pomegranate
- ☐ Raspberries
- ☐ Rhubarb
- ☐ Strawberries
- ☐ Tangerines

Eliminate: dried fruit, fruit juice

ANIMAL PROTEIN

- ☐ Beef
- ☐ Chicken
- ☐ Lamb
- ☐ Pork
- ☐ Turkey

Eliminate: eggs

PLANT PROTEIN

- ☐ Mung bean pasta
- ☐ Nutritional yeast
- ☐ Spirulina

Eliminate: soy (edamame, tempeh, tofu)

UNSWEETENED PROTEIN POWDER

- ☐ Bone broth
- ☐ Collagen peptides
- ☐ Hemp protein
- ☐ Pea protein
- ☐ Rice protein

Eliminate: soy and whey-based protein powders

FISH AND SEAFOOD

- ☐ Crab
- ☐ Fish (salmon, mackerel, anchovies, sardines, herring)
- ☐ Lobster
- ☐ Oysters
- ☐ Prawns
- ☐ Shrimp

UNSWEETENED DAIRY ALTERNATIVES

- [ ] Almond milk
- [ ] Cashew milk
- [ ] Coconut milk
- [ ] Flaxseed milk
- [ ] Hemp milk
- [ ] Macadamia nut milk
- [ ] Rice milk
- [ ] Kefir (such as coconut)
- [ ] Yogurt (such as almond or coconut)

Eliminate: cow's milk/dairy products, goat's milk, soy milk, sweetened yogurts

FROZEN FOODS

- [ ] Frozen fruits
- [ ] Frozen vegetables

GLUTEN-FREE GRAINS

- [ ] Amaranth
- [ ] Buckwheat
- [ ] Millet
- [ ] Quinoa
- [ ] Rice
- [ ] Sorghum
- [ ] Oats (labeled gluten-free)
- [ ] Teff

Eliminate: gluten-containing grains (such as wheat, barley, rye), refined grains (white flour products like bread), corn and corn products (such as chips)

LEGUMES

- [ ] Beans
- [ ] Lentils
- [ ] Peas

Eliminate: peanuts and soy (edamame, tofu, tempeh, soy sauce)

RAW NUTS AND SEEDS

- [ ] All nut butters (except peanut)
- [ ] Almonds
- [ ] Brazil nuts
- [ ] Cashews
- [ ] Chia seeds
- [ ] Coconut
- [ ] Flaxseeds
- [ ] Hemp seeds
- [ ] Macadamia
- [ ] Nut flours (such as almond, coconut)
- [ ] Pecans
- [ ] Pine nuts
- [ ] Pistachios
- [ ] Sesame seeds
- [ ] Sunflower seeds
- [ ] Walnuts

Eliminate: peanuts

FATS AND OILS

- ☐ Avocado
- ☐ Coconut milk
- ☐ Coconut butter
- ☐ Ghee
- ☐ Oils (unrefined, cold-pressed, organic): avocado, coconut, extra-virgin olive oil, flax, hemp, sesame, walnut
- ☐ Olives

Eliminate: highly processed oils (such as canola, corn, soy), margarine, shortening

HERBS, SPICES, CONDIMENTS, MISCELLANEOUS

- ☐ All herbs
- ☐ All spices
- ☐ Coconut aminos
- ☐ Ketchup (unsweetened)
- ☐ Mustard
- ☐ Stevia
- ☐ Vinegars

Eliminate: artificial and natural sweeteners (including aspartame, agave, brown rice syrup, brown sugar, cane sugar, high fructose corn syrup, honey, maple syrup, molasses, saccharin, sucralose, sugar alcohols like xylitol, white sugar), commercial salad dressings, mayonnaise, soy sauce

UNSWEETENED BEVERAGES

- ☐ All teas
- ☐ Bone broth
- ☐ Coffee
- ☐ Matcha
- ☐ Seltzer water

Eliminate: alcohol, energy drinks, fruit juice, sod

CHAPTER 6.2

CANDIDA FOOD PLAN

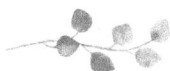

The Candida food plan is designed to get rid of Candida overgrowth by removing the foods that it feeds off of and foods that make symptoms worse. This includes all types of sugar, refined grains, and yeast and mold-containing foods.

Top 5 Foods that Fight Candida

- Coconut oil
- Cinnamon
- Ginger
- Lemon
- Raw garlic

Follow this plan for four weeks. The fifth week, you'll begin the reintroduction phase, which is detailed in Chapter 6.4.

Familiarize yourself with the grocery lists and sample meal

plan included in this chapter. Printable versions are available on my website, renellestayton.com.

EAT	ELIMINATE
Grass-fed meats	All forms of sugar, natural and artificial
Fish and other seafood	White flour products
Eggs	Dairy
Natural fats	Most fermented foods
Low-sugar fruits	High-sugar fruits
Non-starchy vegetables	Starchy vegetables (corn, peas, potatoes, etc.)
Gluten-free whole grains	Vinegars
Legumes (beans, lentils)	Alcohol
Nuts and seeds	Caffeine
All herbs and spices	Yeast and mold containing foods (aged cheeses like blue cheese, baker's yeast, mushrooms, cashews, peanuts, pistachios, etc.)
Stevia	

3-DAY MEAL PLAN

All recipes are listed in the recipe section

	DAY 1	DAY 2	DAY 3
BREAKFAST	Mediterranean Chicken Sausage with Artichoke Dip	Coconut Cinnamon Smoothie	Mediterranean Chicken Sausage with Artichoke Dip
LUNCH	Coconut Curry Soup	Mustard Salmon with Bacon Brussels Sprouts	Coconut Curry Soup
DINNER	Mustard Salmon with Bacon Brussels Sprouts	Coconut Curry Soup	Thai Meatballs with Baby Bok Choy and Rice

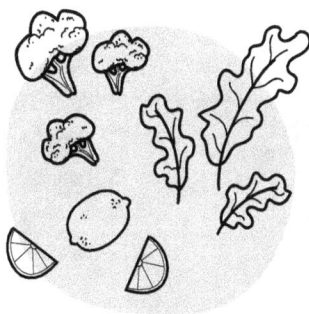

MEAL PLAN GROCERY LIST

VEGETABLES

Non-Starchy

- [ ] Baby bok choy, 6
- [ ] Brussels sprouts, 1 lb
- [ ] Carrots, 3 large
- [ ] Cilantro, 1 bunch
- [ ] Delicata squash, 1
- [ ] Ginger root, 1 large knob
- [ ] Green onions, 2 bunches
- [ ] Parsley, 1 bunch
- [ ] Rutabaga, 1
- [ ] Zucchini, 1

FRUIT

- [ ] Limes, 1
- [ ] Lemons, 2

ANIMAL PROTEIN

- [ ] Ground beef, 1 lb
- [ ] Ground chicken thighs, 1 lb

PLANT PROTEIN

- [ ] Tofu, firm (14 oz)

UNSWEETENED PROTEIN POWDER

- [ ] Vanilla protein powder (bone broth, hemp or soy-based only)

FISH AND SEAFOOD

- [ ] Salmon fillets, 4 (about 6 oz each)

GLUTEN-FREE GRAINS

- [ ] Brown rice

RAW NUTS AND SEEDS

- [ ] Any nuts for snacks (except cashews, peanuts and pistachios)
- [ ] Pumpkin seeds (optional)

FATS AND OILS

- [ ] Extra virgin olive oil
- [ ] Ghee
- [ ] Toasted sesame oil

HERBS, SPICES, CONDIMENTS, MISCELLANEOUS

- [ ] Artichoke hearts, 1 (14 oz) can
- [ ] Bacon, nitrite-free
- [ ] Bone broth, chicken (or any)
- [ ] Cayenne (optional)
- [ ] Cinnamon
- [ ] Coconut aminos
- [ ] Coconut milk, full fat, 2 cans
- [ ] Cumin
- [ ] Dijon mustard
- [ ] Fish sauce (optional)
- [ ] Kalamata olives, pitted
- [ ] Stevia, liquid
- [ ] Tahini
- [ ] Turmeric
- [ ] Za'atar spice

FULL GROCERY LIST

VEGETABLES

Non-Starchy

- ☐ Artichoke
- ☐ Arugula
- ☐ Asparagus
- ☐ Beets
- ☐ Bell peppers
- ☐ Bok choy
- ☐ Broccoli
- ☐ Brussels sprouts
- ☐ Cabbage
- ☐ Carrots
- ☐ Cauliflower
- ☐ Celery
- ☐ Chives
- ☐ Cilantro
- ☐ Cucumber
- ☐ Dill
- ☐ Eggplant
- ☐ Fennel
- ☐ Garlic
- ☐ Green beans
- ☐ Jicama
- ☐ Kale
- ☐ Leeks
- ☐ Lettuce
- ☐ Onion
- ☐ Parsley
- ☐ Radish
- ☐ Rutabaga
- ☐ Shallots
- ☐ Spinach
- ☐ Squash (such as delicata, pumpkin, spaghetti)
- ☐ Swiss chard
- ☐ Tomato
- ☐ Zucchini

Eliminate: fermented vegetables, mushrooms, starchy vegetables (such as corn, peas, potatoes), anything not listed above

FRUIT

Limit to 1 serving per day. Serving size indicated.

- ☐ Apples - 1
- ☐ Apricots - 4
- ☐ Avocado
- ☐ Blackberries - ½ cup
- ☐ Blueberries - ½ cup
- ☐ Cherries - 10
- ☐ Cranberries - ½ cup
- ☐ Figs - 2
- ☐ Grapes - 1 medium bunch
- ☐ Grapefruit - ½ cup
- ☐ Lemons - unlimited
- ☐ Limes - unlimited
- ☐ Nectarine - 1
- ☐ Orange -1
- ☐ Peach - 1
- ☐ Pomegranate seeds - ½ cup
- ☐ Raspberries - 1 cup
- ☐ Rhubarb - 1 cup
- ☐ Strawberries - 1 cup
- ☐ Tangerine - 2

Eliminate: any fruits not listed, dried fruit, fruit juice

ANIMAL PROTEIN

- ☐ Beef
- ☐ Chicken
- ☐ Lamb
- ☐ Pork
- ☐ Turkey
- ☐ Eggs

Eliminate: processed meats (such as hot dogs, sausage)

PLANT PROTEIN

- ☐ Mung bean pasta
- ☐ Spirulina
- ☐ Tempeh
- ☐ Tofu

Eliminate: nutritional yeast

UNSWEETENED PROTEIN POWDER

- ☐ Bone broth
- ☐ Collagen peptides
- ☐ Hemp protein
- ☐ Soy protein

Eliminate: pea and whey-based protein powders

FISH AND SEAFOOD

- ☐ Crab
- ☐ Fish (salmon, mackerel, anchovies, sardines, herring)
- ☐ Lobster
- ☐ Oysters
- ☐ Prawns
- ☐ Shrimp

UNSWEETENED DAIRY ALTERNATIVES

- ☐ Almond milk
- ☐ Cashew milk
- ☐ Coconut milk
- ☐ Hemp milk
- ☐ Soy milk

Eliminate: cow's milk/dairy products, goat's milk, sweetened yogurts

FROZEN FOODS

- ☐ Frozen low-sugar fruits
- ☐ Frozen non-starchy vegetables

GLUTEN-FREE GRAINS

Limit to 1 serving per day. Serving size indicated.

- ☐ Amaranth - ⅓ cup
- ☐ Buckwheat - ½ cup
- ☐ Millet - ½ cup
- ☐ Oats (labeled gluten-free) - ½ cup
- ☐ Pasta - ⅓ cup
- ☐ Quinoa - ½ cup
- ☐ Rice - ⅓ cup
- ☐ Sorghum - ⅓ cup

Eliminate: gluten-containing grains (such as wheat, barley, rye), refined grains (white flour products like bread), corn and corn products (such as chips)

LEGUMES

Limit to 2-3 servings per day. Serving size indicated.

- ☐ Edamame - ½ cup
- ☐ Beans - ½ cup
- ☐ Lentils -½ cup

Eliminate: peas, peanuts

RAW NUTS AND SEEDS

- ☐ Almonds
- ☐ Brazil nuts
- ☐ Chia seeds
- ☐ Coconut
- ☐ Flaxseeds
- ☐ Hemp seeds
- ☐ Macadamia
- ☐ Nut flours (such as almond, coconut)
- ☐ Pecans
- ☐ Pine nuts
- ☐ Sesame seeds
- ☐ Sunflower seeds
- ☐ Walnuts

Eliminate: cashews, peanuts and pistachios

FATS AND OILS

- ☐ Avocado
- ☐ Coconut milk
- ☐ Coconut butter
- ☐ Ghee
- ☐ Oils (unrefined, cold-pressed, organic): avocado, coconut, extra-virgin olive oil, flax, hemp, sesame, walnut
- ☐ Olives

Eliminate: highly processed oils (such as canola, corn, soy), margarine, shortening

HERBS, SPICES, CONDIMENTS, MISCELLANEOUS

- ☐ All herbs
- ☐ All spices
- ☐ Apple cider vinegar
- ☐ Coconut aminos
- ☐ Ketchup (unsweetened)
- ☐ Mustard
- ☐ Stevia

Eliminate: artificial and natural sweeteners (including aspartame, agave, brown rice syrup, brown sugar, cane sugar, high fructose corn syrup, honey, maple syrup, molasses, saccharin, sucralose, sugar alcohols like xylitol, white sugar), commercial salad dressings, soy sauce, all vinegars (except apple cider)

UNSWEETENED BEVERAGES

- ☐ All herbal teas
- ☐ Bone broth
- ☐ Seltzer water

Eliminate: alcohol, caffeinated teas, coffee, energy drinks, fruit juice, soda

CHAPTER 6.3

SIBO FOOD PLAN

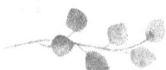

The SIBO food plan is a low-FODMAP diet. FODMAPs are short-chain carbohydrates found in a variety of different foods. FODMAP stands for fermentable oligosaccharides, disaccharides, monosaccharides and polyols.

FODMAPS	EXAMPLES
Oligosaccharides	Fructans and galactooligosaccharides found in wheat, onion, garlic and legumes
Disaccharides	Lactose found in dairy products like milk and cheese
Monosaccharides	Fructose found in apples, honey and high fructose corn syrup
Polyols	Sorbitol and mannitol found in some fruits and vegetables, sugar alcohol sweeteners like xylitol

When you eat FODMAP-containing foods, they're fermented by gut bacteria and can cause gas, bloating and diarrhea—trademark symptoms of SIBO.

Quantity is key when it comes to this diet. Pay attention to serving sizes and their FODMAP content. For example, 12 almonds have a small amount of FODMAPs while 24 have a high amount. I recommend downloading the Monash University FODMAP Diet app as a resource, which outlines the amount of FODMAPs in different quantities of food.

Follow this plan for four weeks. The fifth week, you'll begin the reintroduction phase, which is detailed in Chapter 6.4.

Familiarize yourself with the grocery lists and sample meal plan included in this chapter. Printable versions are available on my website, renellestayton.com.

EAT	ELIMINATE
Grass-fed meats	All forms of sugar, natural and artificial
Fish and other seafood	
Eggs	White flour products
Natural fats	Dairy
Low-FODMAP fruits, vegetables, whole grains, nuts and seeds	Gluten
	Moderate to high-FODMAP vegetables, fruits, whole grains, nuts and seeds
All herbs and spices	
Stevia	Legumes (beans, peas, lentils)
	Alcohol

No Garlic and Onions?

Avoiding garlic and onions is one of the hardest things about eating low-FODMAP. Use chives or the green tops of green onions instead. You can also substitute garlic-infused olive oil in place of regular olive oil, since FODMAPs aren't oil-soluble.

3-DAY MEAL PLAN

All recipes are listed in the recipe section

	DAY 1	DAY 2	DAY 3
BREAKFAST	Mediterranean Chicken Sausage with Artichoke Dip	Coconut Cinnamon Smoothie	Mediterranean Chicken Sausage with Artichoke Dip
LUNCH	Coconut Curry Soup	Mustard Salmon with Baked Sweet Potatoes	Coconut Curry Soup
DINNER	Mustard Salmon with Baked Sweet Potatoes	Coconut Curry Soup	Thai Meatballs with Baby Bok Choy and Rice

MEAL PLAN GROCERY LIST

VEGETABLES

Non–Starchy

- ☐ Baby bok choy, 6
- ☐ Carrots, 3 large
- ☐ Cilantro, 1 bunch
- ☐ Ginger root, 1 large knob
- ☐ Green onions, 2 bunches
- ☐ Parsley, 1 bunch
- ☐ Zucchini, 1

Starchy

- ☐ Sweet potatoes, 4 medium

FRUIT

- ☐ Limes, 1
- ☐ Lemons , 2

ANIMAL PROTEIN

- ☐ Ground beef, 1 lb
- ☐ Ground chicken thighs, 1 lb

PLANT PROTEIN

- ☐ Tofu, firm (14 oz)

UNSWEETENED PROTEIN POWDER

- ☐ Vanilla protein powder (bone broth, hemp or rice-based only)

FISH AND SEAFOOD

- ☐ Salmon fillets, 4 (about 6 oz each)

GLUTEN-FREE GRAINS

- ☐ Brown rice

RAW NUTS AND SEEDS

- ☐ Any nuts for snacks (except cashews, pistachios)
- ☐ Pumpkin seeds (optional)

FATS AND OILS

- ☐ Extra virgin olive oil
- ☐ Ghee
- ☐ Toasted sesame oil

HERBS, SPICES, CONDIMENTS, MISCELLANEOUS

- ☐ Artichoke hearts, 1 (14 oz) can
- ☐ Bone broth, chicken
- ☐ Cayenne (optional)
- ☐ Cinnamon
- ☐ Coconut aminos
- ☐ Coconut milk, full fat, 2 cans (no inulin)
- ☐ Cumin
- ☐ Dijon mustard
- ☐ Fish sauce (optional)
- ☐ Kalamata olives, pitted
- ☐ Stevia, liquid
- ☐ Tahini
- ☐ Turmeric
- ☐ Za'atar spice

FULL GROCERY LIST

Bolded items are moderate to high-FODMAP foods tolerable in smaller amounts (see serving size indicated). Limit these foods to maximum 1 serving from each food category per day.

VEGETABLES

Non-Starchy

- [ ] **Artichoke hearts - ⅛ cup**
- [ ] Arugula
- [ ] Bean sprouts
- [ ] **Beets - ¼ cup**
- [ ] **Bell pepper, red - ¼ cup**
- [ ] Bok choy
- [ ] **Broccoli - ¼ cup**
- [ ] **Cabbage, red - ¼ cup**
- [ ] Carrots
- [ ] **Celery - ¼ stalk**
- [ ] Chives
- [ ] Cilantro
- [ ] Collard greens
- [ ] Cucumber
- [ ] **Eggplant - 1 cup**
- [ ] Fennel
- [ ] **Fermented vegetables (such as sauerkraut) - 1 T**
- [ ] **Green beans, 15**
- [ ] **Green onion (green tops only) - 1 bunch**
- [ ] Kale
- [ ] Lettuce
- [ ] Mushrooms, oyster only - 1 cup
- [ ] Parsley
- [ ] Radish
- [ ] **Spaghetti squash - ½ cup**
- [ ] Spinach
- [ ] Swiss chard
- [ ] Tomato
- [ ] **Zucchini - ⅓ cup**

Starchy

- [ ] Acorn squash
- [ ] **Butternut squash - ¼ cup**
- [ ] **Parsnip - ½ cup**
- [ ] **Potatoes - ½ cup**
- [ ] Plantain
- [ ] **Pumpkin (canned only) - ¾ cup**
- [ ] **Sweet potato - ½ cup**

Eliminate: vegetables not listed above (such as asparagus, Brussels sprouts, cauliflower, corn, garlic, leeks, all mushrooms except oyster, onions, peas, shallots)

FRUIT

- [ ] **Bananas (green/unripe only) - 1 medium**
- [ ] **Blueberries - ¼ cup**
- [ ] **Cantaloupe - ¾ cup**
- [ ] **Clementine - 1 medium**
- [ ] **Grapes - 1 cup**
- [ ] **Kiwi - 2 small**
- [ ] Lemon
- [ ] Lime
- [ ] **Mandarin - 2 small**
- [ ] **Oranges - 1 medium**
- [ ] **Pineapple - 1 cup**
- [ ] **Rhubarb - 1 cup**
- [ ] **Strawberries - 1 cup**

Eliminate: fruits not listed above (such as apples, apricots, avocados, blackberries, cherries, dates, figs, grapefruit, mangos, pears, pomegranate seeds, stone fruits, watermelon), canned fruit, dried fruit, fruit juice

ANIMAL PROTEIN

- ☐ Beef
- ☐ Chicken
- ☐ Lamb
- ☐ Pork
- ☐ Turkey
- ☐ Eggs

PLANT PROTEIN

- ☐ **Edamame - ½ cup**
- ☐ Spirulina
- ☐ **Tempeh - ⅓ cup**
- ☐ **Tofu, firm only- ⅔ cup**

Eliminate: soft/silken tofu

UNSWEETENED PROTEIN POWDER

- ☐ Bone broth
- ☐ Collagen peptides
- ☐ Hemp protein
- ☐ Rice protein

Eliminate: pea, soy and whey-based protein powders

FISH AND SEAFOOD

- ☐ Crab
- ☐ Fish (salmon, mackerel, anchovies, sardines, herring)
- ☐ Lobster
- ☐ Oysters
- ☐ Prawns
- ☐ Shrimp

UNSWEETENED DAIRY ALTERNATIVES

- ☐ Almond milk
- ☐ **Coconut milk, canned (no inulin) - ¼ cup**
- ☐ **Hemp milk - ½ cup**
- ☐ **Macadamia nut milk - 1 cup**
- ☐ **Quinoa milk - 1 cup**
- ☐ **Rice milk - ¼ cup**
- ☐ Yogurt (such as coconut)

Eliminate: cow's milk/dairy products, goat's milk, oat milk, soy milk, sweetened yogurts

FROZEN FOODS

- ☐ Frozen low-FODMAP fruits (see fruit section)
- ☐ Frozen low-FODMAP vegetables (see vegetables section)

GLUTEN-FREE GRAINS

- ☐ **Amaranth - ¼ cup**
- ☐ **Arrowroot powder - ⅔ cup**
- ☐ **Buckwheat - ½ cup**
- ☐ Millet
- ☐ Quinoa
- ☐ Rice
- ☐ Sorghum
- ☐ **Oats - ¼ cup**
- ☐ Teff

Eliminate: gluten-containing grains (such as wheat, barley, rye), refined grains (white flour products like bread)

LEGUMES

Eliminate (most are moderate to high-FODMAP)

RAW NUTS AND SEEDS

- [ ] All nut butters
- [ ] **Almond, tahini - 1 T**
- [ ] **Almonds - 10 nuts**
- [ ] Brazil nuts
- [ ] **Chestnuts - 20 nuts, boiled**
- [ ] **Chia seeds - 2 T**
- [ ] **Coconut (fresh)- ⅓ cup**
- [ ] **Coconut (dried, shredded) - ½ cup**
- [ ] **Flaxseeds - 1 T**
- [ ] Hemp seeds
- [ ] **Macadamia - 20 nuts**
- [ ] Nut Flours
- [ ] **Almond - ¼ cup**
- [ ] Peanuts
- [ ] **Pecans - 10 nuts**
- [ ] **Pine nuts - 1 T**
- [ ] **Sesame seeds - 1 T**
- [ ] **Walnuts - 10 halves**

Eliminate: cashews, hazelnut, coconut flour, pistachios, sunflower seeds

FATS AND OILS

- [ ] Coconut milk (no inulin)
- [ ] Ghee
- [ ] Oils (unrefined, cold-pressed, organic): coconut, extra-virgin olive oil, flax, hemp, sesame, walnut
- [ ] Olives

Eliminate: avocado, highly processed oils (such as canola, corn, soy), margarine, shortening

HERBS, SPICES, CONDIMENTS, MISCELLANEOUS

- [ ] All herbs
- [ ] All spices (except garlic and onion powder)
- [ ] Coconut aminos
- [ ] Ketchup (unsweetened)
- [ ] Mustard
- [ ] Stevia
- [ ] Vinegars (such as apple cider, **balsamic - 1 T**, red wine, white)

Eliminate: artificial and natural sweeteners (including aspartame, agave, brown rice syrup, brown sugar, cane sugar, high fructose corn syrup, honey, maple syrup, molasses, saccharin, sucralose, sugar alcohols like xylitol, white sugar), commercial salad dressings, hummus, garlic and onion powder, soy sauce

UNSWEETENED BEVERAGES

- [ ] All teas (must dilute chai, chamomile and oolong)
- [ ] Bone broth
- [ ] Coffee
- [ ] Matcha
- [ ] Seltzer water

Eliminate: alcohol, energy drinks, fruit juice, soda

CHAPTER 6.4

FOOD REINTRODUCTION

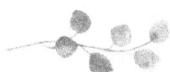

Starting the fifth week, you'll begin to reintroduce the eliminated foods back one-by-one. This chapter outlines how to reintroduce foods for each food plan.

Food reintroduction will tell you what foods to eat and what to not eat after the protocol in order to keep your skin clear. By seeing how your body responds to each food, you'll know whether or not to keep it in your diet. Check in with how you feel before, immediately after, hours after, and days after you've added a new food back in. Your body will tell you what works and what doesn't.

If you have any symptoms, including breakouts, take the food out of your diet. You can try reintroducing it again after you've tested everything else, or wait three months. Some foods you may not want to add back at all.

I recommend continuing to limit your intake of sugar, refined carbohydrates, dairy, gluten and alcohol even after the protocol is over in order to support gut, skin and hormonal health.

SYMPTOM TRACKER

	GLUTEN	DAIRY		
HEADACHE				
CONGESTION				
CONSTIPATION OR **DIARRHEA**				
GAS OR **BLOATING**				
SKIN IRRITATION OR **BLOATING**				
JOINT PAIN				
FATIGUE				
SLEEPINESS AFTER EATING				
SLEEP DISTURBANCE				
OTHER				

FOOD REINTRODUCTION FOR LEAKY GUT

First, decide which food you want to add back into your diet. Choose foods in their purest, simplest forms. For example, if you're reintroducing dairy, try milk—don't eat a cheese pizza, which also contains gluten.

Types of foods to use for reintroduction:

- Gluten - 100% whole wheat noodles
- Dairy - milk, cheese (without additives)
- Egg - soft-boiled or hard-boiled egg, poached egg
- Corn - corn on the cob, plain popcorn
- Soy - edamame, tofu
- Peanuts - plain peanuts
- Natural sugars - honey, maple syrup (add back last)

Eat a serving of the chosen food 2-3 times on the first day, then stop eating it.

- **If you have no reaction after 48 hours, you can now include the food back in your diet.** Reintroduce the next food and repeat the process.

- **If you have a reaction, stop eating the food immediately and do not add it back.** Allow the reaction to clear completely before moving on to reintroducing the next food (this may take several days). Continue to avoid the triggering food until after you've tested all of the other foods. You can reintroduce it at this point or wait three months.

FOOD REINTRODUCTION FOR CANDIDA

Decide which food you want to add back into your diet, then choose a pure and simple form of that food to reintroduce.

Types of foods to use for reintroduction:

- Gluten - 100% whole wheat noodles
- Dairy - milk
- Starchy vegetables, corn - corn on the cob, plain popcorn
- Fermented foods - sauerkraut
- Yeast and mold-containing foods- baker's yeast, aged cheeses like blue cheese
- Natural sugars - honey, maple syrup (add back last)

Eat a serving of the chosen food 2-3 times on the first day, then stop eating it. Notice how you feel before, immediately after, hours after, and days after. Monitor for any type of reaction.

- **If you have no reaction after 48 hours, you can now include the food back in your diet.** Reintroduce the next food and repeat the process.

- **If you have a reaction, stop eating the food immediately and do not add it back.** Allow the reaction to clear completely before moving on to reintroducing the next food (this may take several days). Continue to avoid the triggering food until after you've tested all of the other foods. Then, reintroduce it or wait three months before trying again.

Recurrence of Candida is common. For this reason, it's especially important to limit sugar, refined carbohydrates and certain kinds of alcohol (especially beer and wine) even after you've completed the protocol.

FOOD REINTRODUCTION FOR SIBO

Reintroduce each FODMAP group back into your diet, one-by-one, while continuing to keep your background diet low-FODMAP. You'll eat increasing amounts of the FODMAP group over a period of three days, followed by a "washout" period.

Monitor for any type of reactions.

DAY 1	Eat a small serving (¼ normal serving) of the FODMAP group • If you have no symptoms: go to day 2 • If you have symptoms: this group is a trigger for you. Stop eating the FODMAP group and start the washout period.
DAY 2	Eat a medium serving (½ normal serving) of the FODMAP group • If you have no symptoms: go to day 3 • If you have symptoms: you can tolerate small amounts of this FODMAP group (¼ normal serving). You can add this amount back into your long-term diet. Start the washout period before adding the next FODMAP group.

Continued on following page

DAY 3	Eat a full serving of the FODMAP group. • If you have no symptoms: you can add the FODMAP group back into your long-term diet. • If you have symptoms: you can tolerate medium amounts (½ normal serving) of this FODMAP group. You can add this amount back into your long-term diet. Start the washout period before adding the next FODMAP group.
WASHOUT PERIOD	Take 2-3 days (or longer) to clear any symptoms. Wait until all symptoms disappear before reintroducing the next FODMAP group.

FODMAP Groups for Reintroduction

- Galactooligosaccharides: almonds
  - ▸ Day 1: 5 nuts = ¼ serving
  - ▸ Day 2: 10 nuts = ½ serving
  - ▸ Day 3: 20 nuts = 1 full serving

- Lactose: yogurt (evaluates dairy tolerance as well)
  - ▸ Day 1: 4 oz
  - ▸ Day 2: 8 oz
  - ▸ Day 3: 12 oz

- Fructose: honey
  - Day 1: ¾ tsp = ¼ serving
  - Day 2: 1½ tsp = ½ serving
  - Day 3: 1 T = 1 full serving

- Fructans: 100% whole wheat bread (evaluates gluten tolerance as well)
  - Day 1: ½ a slice = ¼ serving
  - Day 2: 1 slice = ½ serving
  - Day 3: 2 slices = 1 full serving

- Polyols, Mannitol: sweet potato
  - Day 1: 2 T = ¼ serving
  - Day 2: ¼ cup = ½ serving
  - Day 3: ½ cup = 1 full serving

- Polyols, Sorbitol: avocado
  - Day 1: 2 T = ¼ serving
  - Day 2: ¼ avocado = ½ serving
  - Day 3: ½ avocado = 1 full serving

Recurrence of SIBO is common. To help prevent this, support proper functioning of the migrating motor complex (MMC) by spacing meals at least 4-5 hours apart and fasting for 12 hours overnight. Consider using promotility agents (also known as prokinetics) which stimulate the cleansing waves of the MMC. Examples include: ginger, Swedish bitters, bitter greens and fennel seeds.

SUMMARY

The fifth week of the protocol, you'll reintroduce eliminated foods back into your diet one by one. Notice how your skin and body react to each food that you add back. Certain foods may make you break out or feel fatigued, while other foods continue to make your skin look radiant and give you energy. This is all valuable information because it enables you to personalize your diet to maintain clear skin after the protocol.

Key takeaways

- You can try retesting foods that you had a reaction to *after* you've tested everything else, or you can continue to keep them out of your diet

- Continue to limit intake of sugar, refined carbohydrates, dairy, gluten and alcohol even after the protocol to support gut, skin and hormonal health

CHAPTER 7

SUPPLEMENTS

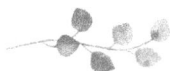

Baseline supplements are used to support overall health. Multivitamins and omega-3s help correct underlying nutrient deficiencies which contribute to acne, while digestive enzymes and betaine HCL aid digestion and absorption of nutrients. It can be difficult to get enough nutrients from diet alone, due to factors like nutrient-depleted soil and increasing reliance on genetically modified foods.

In addition to the baseline supplements, targeted supplement therapy for each gut condition is also included. These supplements help heal a damaged gut barrier or "weed out" overgrowth of Candida or SIBO.

Supplements (nutritional, herbal or otherwise) can have different effects on different people. Any supplement can have side effects and can interact with medications or other supplements that you're taking. Consult with your healthcare provider before taking anything new.

High-quality brands I recommend:

- Thorne
- Pure Encapsulations
- Metagenics
- Nordic Naturals
- Klaire Labs
- Designs for Health
- Integrative Therapeutics

You can purchase products directly from the brand websites or find them at your local health food store. For quality assurance, look to see if the product has the National Sanitation Foundation (NSF) certification or the U.S. Pharmacopeial Convention (USP) verification on their label (or your country's equivalent).

BASELINE SUPPLEMENTS

SUPPLEMENTS	DOSE
Multivitamin, high-quality	Take as directed by manufacturer
Omega-3s, fish oil (purified)	2 grams EPA/DHA daily
Digestive enzymes	1-2 capsules, with meals

Betaine HCL	First, do the baking soda or betaine HCL test (outlined under betaine HCL section). If you need to take it, take your specific dose with protein-rich meals.

Why are these important for skin health?

MULTIVITAMIN

Multivitamins are a practical and cost-effective way to meet baseline nutrient needs. Rather than buying individual supplements, multivitamins contain a blend of vitamins and minerals that are important for healing acne and beneficial for overall health.

Vitamins and minerals that heal acne:

- Vitamin A
- B vitamins (such as B3, B5)
- Vitamin C
- Vitamin D3
- Vitamin E
- Zinc

Read the label to see how many capsules are in one serving. It can be anywhere from 1-8 capsules, depending on the brand.

What to look for in a multivitamin

- **Vitamin D3, not D2.** Vitamin D3 is the more biologically active form of vitamin D.

- **Folate, not folic acid.** Folic acid is the synthetic form of folate. Look for folate instead, which can also be listed as "5-methyltetrahydrofolate" or "5-MTHF". Certain people with MTHFR gene variants can't effectively process folic acid so this distinction is important.

- **At least 15-30mg of zinc.** Zinc helps the skin turnover and prevents acne from developing. People with acne have been found to have lower levels of zinc in their blood and skin [1-3]. Studies have found that supplementing with zinc is as effective as tetracycline antibiotics at treating acne [4]. Look for a multivitamin that has between 15-30mg of zinc, depending on how much you're getting from dietary sources. Avoid long-term supplementation with doses >40mg/day, which can result in copper deficiency.

Vitamin D Testing

Vitamin D deficiency is very common. Having adequate vitamin D levels helps fight inflammation that contributes to acne. Your body produces this vitamin when you expose your skin to natural sunlight. If you spend most of your time indoors, overuse sunscreen, live in a northern climate or have darker skin, this can affect your body's production of vitamin D. It's a good idea to have your level checked with a blood test called the 25-hydroxy vitamin D test. An optimal level is >40ng/mL.

OMEGA-3S

Healthy fats are critical for cellular function. All cells in your body have fatty acids that help hold them together. Fatty acids, like omega-3s and omega-6s, are considered "essential" because your body can't make them on its own—you have to get them from your diet.

Remember: you are what you eat. Most people in westernized countries get about a 20:1 ratio of omega-6s to omega-3s, which promotes inflammation. You want this ratio to be closer to 4:1.

Omega-6s are found in plant-based oils, such as refined canola, corn and soybean oils. They're cheaper to produce than oils like olive oil, which is why they're added to virtually all processed foods, like commercial salad dressings, chips and fast food. While omega-6s from high quality sources are important for health, too many omega-6s from poor quality sources can contribute to obesity, depression and inflammatory disorders.

Omega-3s play a major role in lowering inflammation [5]. Most people are deficient in omega-3s, including people with acne. Supplementation with omega-3s significantly decreased acne lesions in one 10-week randomized, double-blind, controlled trial [6].

There are ways to test your omega-3 levels, like doing an omega-3 index test, but you can also survey your diet to see if you're consuming enough from food sources (like salmon and flaxseeds) on a regular basis. If it seems like you're not getting enough from diet alone, consider supplementing.

DIGESTIVE ENZYMES

There's no point in eating a healthy diet if you can't properly absorb it. Digestive enzymes help your body do this. They contain things like protease to help break down proteins, lipase to break down fats and amylase to break down complex carbohydrates.

BETAINE HCL

Betaine HCL is a supplemental form of stomach acid. Your stomach needs acid to be healthy and many people have stomach acid levels that are too low. This problem is exacerbated if you take drugs like acid-blockers, which block (or decrease) the production of stomach acid.

Without enough stomach acid, you can't break down proteins and vitamin B12, activate digestive enzymes, or protect your gut against infections. Low stomach acid is also a major underlying cause of SIBO.

Symptoms associated with having high stomach acid, like heartburn, are often a sign that you have low stomach acid. This is because low stomach acid causes pressure changes in the gut that allow small amounts of stomach acid to travel back up into your esophagus, causing heartburn.

There are two tests you can do to figure out if you have low stomach acid. The first test is the baking soda test, which isn't as accurate, but is free and easy to do at home. Alternatively, you can do the betaine HCL test, which involves taking betaine HCL to see if it provokes any symptoms of heartburn. This test is contra-indicated if you have peptic ulcer disease, acute gastritis or are taking drugs like NSAIDs or acid-blockers.

BAKING SODA TEST

1. Mix ¼ tsp baking soda into a small glass of water. Drink it first thing in the morning on an empty stomach.

- If you belch within 5 minutes, your stomach acid levels are sufficient. You don't need to do the betaine HCL test or supplement with betaine HCL.

- If you don't belch within 5 minutes, your stomach acid levels are probably low and you should do the betaine HCL test to see how much you should supplement with.

BETAINE HCL TEST

1. Take one capsule (about 650 mg) of betaine HCL with a protein-rich meal. For the next 30 minutes, monitor for any signs of heartburn.

   - If you **do** experience heartburn, then you likely have adequate stomach acid levels. You don't need to take betaine HCL.

   - If you **don't** experience heartburn, your stomach acid levels are probably low and you'll need to supplement with betaine HCL. Take two capsules of betaine HCL with your next protein-rich meal and monitor for heartburn. If you experience heartburn with two capsules, decrease your dose back to one capsule for the remainder of the protocol. You can continue testing until you reach a max of three capsules. Continue betaine HCL for 4-8 weeks. You can wean off of it as your body is able to maintain adequate HCL levels over time.

SUPPLEMENTS FOR LEAKY GUT

SUPPLEMENT	DOSE
Baseline supplements	
Probiotics	10-20 billion CFUs daily Take for one month or longer if needed
L-glutamine	1-3 grams daily Take for one month or longer if needed
Demulcent herbs (DGL, marshmallow root, slippery elm)	Take as directed by manufacturer Take for one month or longer if needed Example: GI-Encap by Thorne

Why are these important for leaky gut?

PROBIOTICS

Probiotics restore balance to the microbiome, especially if you've taken antibiotics. They also decrease skin inflammation, lower oxidative stress markers and improve insulin sensitivity [7-10].

There are significant gut microbiome changes in people with acne compared to healthy controls. People with acne have lower levels of certain beneficial bacterial species (like Bifidobacterium and Lactobacillus) as well as distinct differences in microbiome diversity [11,12].

Look for probiotics that contain Lactobacillus rhamnosus or Bifidobacterium bifidum, which are beneficial for skin health, and keep your probiotics refrigerated.

L-GLUTAMINE AND/OR DEMULCENT HERBS

L-glutamine is an amino acid that provides fuel for intestinal cells, stimulates cell growth of the gut barrier, regulates tight junctions and decreases inflammation [13,14].

Demulcent herbs, such as deglycyrrhizinated licorice (DGL), marshmallow root and slippery elm, soothe inflamed gut tissue by forming a protective mucus-like film called "mucilage". Use them along with L-glutamine to heal your gut barrier.

SUPPLEMENTS FOR CANDIDA

SUPPLEMENT	DOSE
Baseline supplements	
Caprylic acid	800mg twice daily, on an empty stomach Take for one month Example: Caprylic Acid by Pure Encapsulations

Why is this important for Candida?

CAPRYLIC ACID

Caprylic acid is a medium-chain fatty acid found in tropical oils like coconut oil. It's a natural anti-fungal that breaks down yeast cell membranes.

SUPPLEMENTS FOR SIBO

SUPPLEMENT	DOSE
Baseline supplements	
Herbal antibiotic blend containing things like berberine, oregano oil and/or wormwood	Dosing depends on product being used Take for one month Example: Candibactin-BR and Candibactin-AR by Metagenics, taken together. Take as directed by the manufacturer.

Why is this important for SIBO?

HERBAL ANTIBIOTICS

Herbal antibiotics are a gentler and natural alternative to antibiotic drugs. They help "weed out" the bacterial overgrowth in your small intestine. Studies have found that herbal antibiotics (such as the Candibactin-BR and Candibactin-AR products) are as effective as the antibiotic rifaximin at treating SIBO [15].

Don't take these for longer than one to two months. You want to avoid undue stress on the regular healthy bacteria in your gut and you don't want to overburden your liver, which has to metabolize and detoxify any die-off.

Berberine is a chemical compound found in plants like goldenseal, barberry and tree turmeric. It has broad antibacterial activities, regulates blood sugar, improves insulin sensitivity and reduces inflammation [15-17]. Oregano oil and wormwood have well-documented antibacterial effects which help eradicate SIBO [18,19].

SUMMARY

Supplements can correct nutrient deficiencies and restore gut health.

Key takeaways

- Baseline supplements: multivitamin, omega-3s, digestive enzymes and betaine HCL

- Determine if stomach acid level is low with baking soda test or betaine HCL test

- Supplement with betaine HCL only if indicated

- Supplements for leaky gut: probiotics, L-glutamine and/or demulcent herbs

- Supplements for Candida: caprylic acid

- Supplements for SIBO: herbal antibiotic blends containing things like berberine, oregano oil and/or wormwood (example: Candibactin-BR and Candibactin-AR by Metagenics)

CHAPTER 8

TOPICAL TREATMENTS

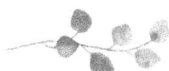

According to the Environmental Working Group (EWG), on average, women use 12 personal care products with 168 different chemicals every day. Men use six products, with 85 different chemicals daily.

What about you?

Personal Care Products

- Face wash
- Toner
- Serum
- Moisturizer
- Sunscreen
- Chapstick
- Makeup
- Deodorant

Continued on following page

- Lotion
- Perfume
- Shampoo
- Conditioner
- Body wash
- Shaving cream
- Hand soap
- Hand sanitizer

It's easy to see how this number can add up quickly!

KNOW YOUR INGREDIENTS

Personal care products are not tightly regulated in countries like the United States. The U.S. Food and Drug Administration (FDA) doesn't require safety testing of many of the chemical ingredients, so ingredients like formaldehyde, mercury, parabens and triclosan (that have been banned by more than 40 countries) are still routinely added to personal care products. This is troubling from a healthcare standpoint, as these chemicals have been associated with cancer and reproductive and neurologic harm [1-3].

How can something that goes on top of your skin cause problems? **Well, your skin isn't a waterproof raincoat—it's more like a sponge.** What you put on it gets absorbed and goes into your bloodstream (that's how things like the birth control patch work).

It can be overwhelming to figure out what ingredients are safe and what should be avoided. Use the EWG Skin Deep database (ewg.org/skindeep) to help you find products that have clean, non-toxic ingredients. You can also look for the green EWG label on products.

What are Clean, Natural Ingredients?

Clean, means "non-toxic". Natural refers to ingredients that are derived from nature, including things like plants, honey, clay, vitamins and minerals. The best way to know what's in your products is to look at the ingredient list on the back. Use the Skin Deep database to help you, too. Don't be fooled by pretty packaging or labels that say "natural"—it's an unregulated term that's just a marketing buzzword.

Don't worry if you can't find the "perfect" product. To help you, I've included product examples for each skincare step.

Avoid these harmful ingredients:

- **Anything with fragrance or parfum.** Fragrance brands don't have to disclose their "secret formulas", which means that fragrances can contain hundreds of chemicals (many of which trigger allergic reactions and breakouts).

- **Formaldehyde and formaldehyde releasers.** These are used as preservatives and help prevent bacterial growth. They've been linked to sun sensitivity and cancer. You can find them in nail polish, body wash, hair products and eye shadows.

- **Oxybenzone.** This is used in some sunscreens to block UV light. It harms coral reefs and marine life and is a hormone disruptor.

- **Parabens.** These are used as preservatives in many cosmetics and skincare products. They're associated with hormone disruption and obesity.

- **Phthalates.** These are added to fragrances to make them stay longer on the skin. They're known hormone disruptors and are associated with decreased fertility.

- **Sodium lauryl sulfate (SLS).** This surfactant is found in cleansers, body washes and mascara. When it combines with other chemicals, it forms carcinogenic compounds.

- **Triclosan.** This is found in antibacterial hand soaps and hand sanitizers. It's a known skin irritant and hormone disruptor.

THE CLEAN SKINCARE ROUTINE

While diet, supplements and lifestyle habits provide the foundation for clear skin, topical treatments (AKA your skincare products) are added in to help shift your skin towards its optimal state.

I'm guessing that whatever topical medications you're using aren't working (or you wouldn't be reading this book). The goal is for you to not have to use any topical medications, so if you're ready, transition to this skincare routine instead.

The guidelines are simple:

- Use less products
- Use less ingredients
- Choose clean, natural ingredients
- Choose eco-friendly products when possible
- Avoid allergens and irritants (fragrances, dyes, alcohols, most essential oils)

Pretty straightforward, right?

When you're always adding new products into your skincare routine, the new product has the potential to interact with or block the action of another product. When you use less products, which usually means less ingredients, you're removing as many potential triggers for your acne as possible. It's like an elimination diet for your skincare routine.

What you don't put on your face is just as important as what you do put on it!

Remember to patch test anything new before using it all over your face. Refer to Chapter 4 for instructions on how to do this.

So, let's get to it. Here's the clean skincare routine:

CLEANSE	Gentle cleanser with clean, natural ingredients (<10 ingredients ideal)
TREAT	Niacinamide (vitamin B3)
MOISTURIZE	Rosehip seed oil

Optional add-ons

TONER	Apple cider vinegar, diluted, once or twice weekly
FACE MASK	Aloe vera matcha or manuka honey cinnamon mask, once weekly
MAKEUP	Mineral makeup
PROTECT	Broad-spectrum, natural sunscreen, as needed

I know that asking you to try a new skincare routine can be scary.

Trust me—I used to think natural skincare products were pretty worthless. How could something natural be more effective than medication? (Yet, ironically, my medications weren't doing anything to fix my skin).

I stuck with the same six skincare products for years. Years! While I may have seen an initial improvement when I first started using them, that tiny glimmer of hope made me decide that they were "safe" to use forever. Using so many products with harsh ingredients made my skin very sensitive and prone to breakouts, especially if I added in anything new.

After training in functional medicine and making major changes to my diet and lifestyle, I knew that upgrading my skincare routine was *way* overdue. I started looking into the research about natural topical therapies for acne, soon realizing that some of the natural therapies were just as effective as acne medications.

Over time, I simplified my skincare routine, made sure my

products had as few ingredients as possible, switched to natural acne treatments, traded regular makeup for mineral makeup and stopped wearing makeup every day. And guess what? **My skin has never looked better.**

I'm asking you to *do less* so you can see how beautiful your skin is when you don't interfere with its natural processes. Harsh topicals disrupt your skin as it tries to rebalance itself. Do you really think that something that bleaches fabric is the best option for your skin? Probably not.

If you still need convincing, here are some other things to consider:

- You're building a foundation for clear skin with diet, supplements and lifestyle habits. Your topical treatments are *complementary* to this. Once the cleanup is done inside of your body, the outside will reflect it.

- You're approaching your skincare routine like a science experiment. You're removing as many potential variables as possible, patch testing products beforehand, adjusting your routine based on careful monitoring, and using what works best for *your* skin—not anyone else's.

- You're supporting your skin's natural flora rather than continually wiping it out with harsh topicals like antibiotics or benzoyl peroxide.

- You're layering products in the correct order to maximize their effectiveness.

- You don't have to guess what products to use in your skincare routine.

Now, let's take a look at each of the skincare steps in detail. They're listed in the order that you would apply them. Omit any of the optional steps that you're not doing.

Cleanse

Use a gentle cleanser with clean, natural ingredients and less than 10 ingredients if possible. Look at the ingredient list to see what's in your cleanser before buying it.

Avoid harsh surfactants like sodium lauryl sulfate (SLS) which are often added to cleansers. While these surfactants are good at getting rid of dirt, they disrupt the delicate structure of the outermost skin layer, called the stratum corneum. They strip away important lipids, proteins and natural moisturizing factor (NMF) components, leading to dry, irritated skin that's prone to breakouts.

Cleanse your face once at night before bed. That's it. You don't want to overwash your face because it strips the skin of its natural oils (which makes your skin produce *more* oil) and can be irritating. However, you do want to rinse off your face if you've been sweating a lot, like after workouts.

CLEANSING METHOD

1. Wash your hands. Remove any makeup with a make-up remover wipe.

2. Rinse your face with warm water (never hot).

3. Lather a small amount of cleanser all over your face.

4. Gently massage it onto your face using small circular motions.

5. Rinse off the lather with warm water. Pat your face dry with a clean towel.

- Naturally Clear Cleansing Foam - Metabolic Maintenance
- Gentle Cleansing Gel - Live Botanical

Tone - optional

Use this toner after cleansing, once or twice per week. Mix 1 part apple cider vinegar (ACV) with 3 parts water. Put the toner into a spray bottle and spray it onto a cotton round before swiping it over your face. Let it sit for one minute, then rinse it off. Don't apply ACV undiluted onto your skin.

ACV is made from fermented apple cider. It contains organic acids—like acetic, citric, lactic and malic acids—that have exfoliating effects when applied topically and a naturally acidic pH to help balance the pH of the outermost skin layer. Some of the acids exhibit antibacterial activity against the bacteria associated with acne and have been found to improve both dry and oily skin [4-7]. Use organic apple cider vinegar that contains the mother.

Treat

Niacinamide, also known as nicotinamide, is a form of vitamin B3 that has numerous skin benefits. It regulates sebum production, reduces redness and hyperpigmentation, improves the appearance of pores and is anti-inflammatory [8,9]. Clinical trials comparing 4% niacinamide and 1% clindamycin (a topical antibiotic prescribed for acne) found that niacinamide is as effective as the antibiotic at treating acne [10,11].

Use niacinamide as a leave-on acne treatment. You can apply it before your moisturizer or look for moisturizers that include it as an ingredient.

• Naturally Clear Topical Spray - Metabolic Maintenance

Moisturize

Botanical oils deliver skin-healing nutrients directly onto the skin and help maintain the integrity of the skin barrier. Rosehip seed oil comes from the bright red seed pods of roses and is ideal for acne-prone skin. It's considered a dry oil, which means that it readily absorbs into the skin and doesn't leave behind a heavy oily residue.

Benefits of this oil are that it contains tretinoin, a type of retinoid that fights acne, and antioxidants like vitamin C, which combat hyperpigmentation. Rosehip seed oil is also high in linoleic acid, which people with acne have been found to have lower levels of in their skin [12]. Low linoleic acid causes sebum to be stickier and increases breakouts.

It can be an adjustment for your skin to use oil alone, so I recommend phasing it in. **To start, mix 1-2 drops of rosehip seed oil with a regular moisturizer.** See how your skin responds to it. Eventually, you can use less/no moisturizer and up to 3-4 drops of oil, or continue to use a combination of the two. I found that it took several weeks for my skin to adjust to using just oil.

Look for organic, cold-pressed and sustainably harvested oils whenever possible. Oils should be packaged in dark bottles to preserve their quality.

EXAMPLES

• Rosehip seed oil - Mountain Rose Herbs

What About Other Oils?

Cannabidiol (CBD) oil is also beneficial for acne. It's made by extracting CBD from cannabis leaves and diluting it in a carrier oil, like jojoba or rosehip seed oil. When applied topically, CBD delivers nutrients (like vitamins A and D) that support skin cell growth and aid in skin repair. It's also anti-inflammatory and decreases sebum production [13].

I recommend not using coconut or olive oil on your face unless you know that your skin already tolerates it. While they may be beneficial for other skin types, they are usually too heavy for acne-prone skin.

When shopping for a regular moisturizer, look for the following ingredients:

- Aloe vera
- Ceramides
- Components of the skin's natural moisturizing factors (NMF), like sodium PCA
- Glycerin
- Hyaluronic acid
- Manuka honey

Like you did with your cleanser, look for a moisturizer with clean, natural ingredients and as few ingredients as possible.

EXAMPLES

- Tolérance Extrême Emulsion - Avène

Face mask - optional

These are optional face masks that you can do once per week. Choose the mask that best suits your skin type.

ALOE VERA MATCHA FACE MASK

For normal, combination or oily skin

Aloe vera gel contains sulfur and salicylic acid, which are common ingredients found in acne treatments. Matcha powder is rich in polyphenols, like EGCG, which reduce sebum, fight inflammation and have anti-wrinkle activity [14-16].

Ingredients

- 2 tsp aloe vera gel, fresh or store-bought (look for preservative-free)
- ¼ tsp matcha powder

Directions

1. Cleanse your face.
2. Mash the aloe gel with a fork and whisk it together with the matcha powder. It's okay if there's still a few big chunks of the aloe gel leftover.

3. Apply the mask to your face and leave it on for 15 minutes.

4. Rinse off with warm water. Pat your face dry and apply moisturizer afterwards.

How to Harvest Aloe Gel

Make sure your plant has a few strong leaves first. Cut off a large leaf at the base, then slice the stalk in half. Scoop out the clear gel inside with a spoon. If you're harvesting more than ¼ cup, you can purée it in a food processor (or blender) to get rid of the big chunks. Fresh aloe gel can be stored in the refrigerator for one month.

MANUKA HONEY CINNAMON FACE MASK

For dry skin

When used together, honey and cinnamon fight bacteria involved in acne [17].

Manuka honey is produced by bees that feed off of the manuka tree, which is native to Australia and New Zealand. It is a natural humectant (meaning it draws in and retains moisture) and has four times the amount of nutrients that regular honey does. Manuka nectar contains a compound that is converted to something called methylglyoxal. If there is more methylglyoxal, it means that the manuka honey is more antibacterial. There is a rating scale that measures this called the Unique Manuka Factor (UMF). Look for manuka honey with a UMF rating of 15 or more to use on your skin.

Cinnamon contains cinnamaldehyde and cinnamic acid, which have antibacterial, anti-inflammatory and antioxidant effects. Topical application of cinnamon gel has been found to significantly reduce acne lesions and decrease skin redness [18].

Ingredients

- 1 tsp manuka honey
- ¼ tsp cinnamon

Directions

1. Cleanse your face.

2. Mix the manuka honey and cinnamon together in a small bowl.

3. Apply the mask to your face and leave it on for 15 minutes.

4. Before rinsing off, lightly tap areas of your skin where there's congestion and breakouts. **Honey-tapping helps draw out sebum and other impurities from your pores.**

5. Rinse off with warm water. Pat your face dry and apply moisturizer afterwards.

Protect – as needed

Look for a broad-spectrum, natural sunscreen without harmful chemicals. I've always had a problem with sunscreens breaking me out, so I'll sometimes wear protective clothing and limit exposure during peak sun hours instead. Use your judgment here.

Makeup - optional

Switch to mineral-based makeup and wear makeup as little as possible. Mineral makeup is made from earth minerals. It contains fewer ingredients than other kinds of makeup and is usually free from artificial colors, oils, fragrances and preservatives that can be problematic for acne-prone skin. When applied, it sits on top of the skin (so it won't clog pores) and creates a natural barrier against environmental factors. It also has the added benefit of sun protection, due to ingredients like zinc oxide.

SAMPLE MAKEUP ROUTINE

1. Mineral foundation, which doubles as a concealer (mix a small amount of foundation powder with a drop of rosehip oil and dab onto blemishes as cover-up)
2. Mineral eyeshadow, eyeliner, mascara
3. Natural lightweight lip balm

Less is more. Layering too many products on top of your skin can create more problems, like *acne cosmetica*—a type of acne triggered by cosmetics. For now, try to avoid any extra makeup steps unless it's for a special occasion.

Examples

• Annmarie

SUMMARY

Follow the general guidelines: use less products, use less ingredients, choose clean and natural ingredients, choose eco-friendly products when possible and avoid potential allergens and irritants (fragrances, dyes, alcohols, most essential oils).

Key takeaways

- Use the EWG Skin Deep database to help you choose clean products
- Use a gentle cleanser with clean, natural ingredients (<10 ingredients ideal)
- Treat with niacinamide (vitamin B3)
- Moisturize with rosehip seed oil, with or without a regular moisturizer
- Optional: tone with diluted apple cider vinegar, once or twice weekly
- Optional: aloe vera matcha or manuka honey cinnamon face mask, once weekly
- If you wear makeup, switch to mineral-based makeup and wear makeup as little as possible

CHAPTER 9

LIFESTYLE HACKS

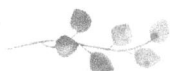

Designing your lifestyle to optimize overall health has a huge impact on your skin.

FIVE MINUTES OF MEDITATION

Mindfulness practices like meditation are a proven way to manage stress. While mindfulness can be practiced in any part of your life—like walking outside, playing an instrument, or even eating—I find that taking the time to quietly sit and meditate is one of the most powerful healing tools. Sitting still, slowing your breathing, and bringing your attention to the present moment has the effect of rewiring your stress response, calming your nervous system and healing your skin [1].

There's no such thing as a "good" or "bad" meditation. **I recommend sitting in meditation for at least five minutes every day.** You can do anything for five minutes! Work your way up to longer time intervals as you're able.

Loving-Kindness Meditation Exercise

Loving-kindness meditation, also known as "metta" meditation, is where you repeat phrases of well-wishes towards yourself or others. Directing the good intentions towards yourself is especially important for acne-sufferers.

This exercise may feel soothing or even uncomfortable—it depends on where you are right now. Sometimes when you feel grief or anger, it can indicate that your heart is softening to reveal what is underneath.

Sit in a comfortable position with your eyes closed, placing one hand over your heart. Recite the following in your mind:

May I be happy
May I be healthy
May I be safe
May I be at peace

Focus on your breath as you feel it move through your chest, filling your heart. Let the intention of the words sink in. Repeat.

Rewrite the Script

Louise Hay, author of *Heal Your Body*, writes that acne is a symptom of not accepting the self or dislike of the self. She suggests replacing the negative thought pattern with a new one: that you love and accept yourself where you are right now. Next time you're tempted to criticize yourself, replace it with "I love and accept myself" instead. This shift in mindset is deeply healing on a cellular level.

Silent Meditation Exercise

Find a comfortable cross-legged position, or sit upright in a chair, resting your palms comfortably on your knees. Sit up tall through your spine and soften your shoulders away from your ears. Close your eyes. Take a slow, deep breath in and out through your nose, bringing your attention to your inhale and exhale. Continue breathing and bringing your attention back to your breath.

You may notice that your mind is wandering—that's normal. Acknowledge the thoughts before gently bringing your attention back to your breath.

SLEEP

There's a reason why it's called beauty sleep! Your skin is fighting off constant attacks during the day and is in "protect" mode. During the night, it switches to "repair and regenerate" mode. Skin regeneration can be up to three times faster at night compared to daytime.

As the sleep hormone melatonin begins to rise in the evening, it offsets damage from things like air pollution and UV radiation, while another hormone, called human growth hormone (HGH), increases cell turnover and accelerates skin repair. The temperature of your skin rises as you sleep, making it more receptive to whatever is left on it or put on it. That's why removing old makeup and applying nourishing products at bedtime is best. Using products like moisturizers also counteracts the transepidermal water loss that occurs in the early morning, which can leave your skin dry and prone to irritation.

Aside from skin health, sleep is also essential for memory and cognition, weight management, mood regulation, energy and immune function. The brain's waste removal system, called the glymphatic system, can only rid itself of waste if you are getting deep and restful sleep.

Aim for eight hours of sleep every night.

Tips for better sleep

- Go to bed and wake up at the same time every day, including weekends
- Keep your room cool (between 60-67°F) and dark
- Use a blackout curtain
- Avoid electronics at least an hour before bed
- Install a blue-light filter on your phone and computer
- Exercise regularly
- Eat your last meal at least three hours before bed
- Avoid drinking caffeine after 12pm
- Switch to tea instead of coffee
- Avoid alcohol, which can interfere with sleep and dehydrate your skin

Bedtime Tea

- 1 part chamomile
- 1 part lemon balm

Directions

1. Combine herbs. Use 2 tsp of mixed herbs per 8 oz of water.

2. Steep herbs for 10 minutes in boiling water, covered. This helps to preserve the medicinal oils from the herbs.

3. Drink tea at least an hour before bedtime.

HORMONAL BREAKOUTS

Testing for hormonal imbalance first is recommended to guide treatment.

Androgen excess and spearmint tea

If you have excess androgens, as seen in polycystic ovarian syndrome (PCOS), consider drinking two cups of spearmint tea daily. Spearmint tea has anti-androgen effects, decreasing testosterone levels that contribute to hormonal acne [2,3]. Spironolactone, a drug prescribed for hormonal acne, is an anti-androgen.

I recommend the spearmint tea by Traditional Medicinals. Steep the tea in boiling water for at least 10 minutes, covered, before drinking. If you are allergic to mint (or related plants like basil, oregano and rosemary) you'll want to skip this tea.

Estrogen dominance and DIM

If you're struggling with estrogen dominance, consider supplementing with diindolylmethane (DIM). DIM is a phytonutrient found in cruciferous vegetables like broccoli, cauliflower, kale and radishes. You'd have to eat about ten pounds of broccoli to get a therapeutic amount of DIM, so supplementing is preferable.

DIM helps your liver increase the amount of "good" estrogen metabolites instead of the "bad". It also inhibits the enzyme aromatase from converting testosterone to estrogen, which can make estrogen dominance worse.

Take 100mg of DIM daily. It can take up to three months to notice a change in your skin, so give it time. Discontinue taking DIM if you experience any negative side effects, common side effects are headache and nausea. It can decrease the efficacy of certain medications, so consult with your healthcare provider before taking it.

Other things that help with estrogen dominance:

- Get enough fiber in your diet, 30-50 grams daily
- Avoid industrial meat and dairy products
- Drink filtered water
- Lose excess body weight
- Make sure you're pooping at least 1-2 times daily
- Create space to de-stress using meditation, yoga, gratitude, etc.

DETOX YOUR HOME

The primary goal here is to decrease your toxic burden, which helps clear your skin. Make small, incremental and budget-friendly choices as you see fit.

- Use natural, unscented cleaning products
- Swap out plastic for glass food containers
- Use a high-quality water filter for drinking and bathing
- Keep windows open to ventilate your home
- Buy more house plants to help filter air
- Use natural weed or pest killers
- Test for and address issues with environmental molds and mycotoxins
- Use essential oil diffusers instead of air fresheners with artificial scents
- Minimize electromagnetic field (EMF) exposure, keep phones in airplane mode at night
- Invest in a non-toxic, organic mattress and bedding

DIY All-Purpose Cleaner

- 2 cups water
- ½ cup distilled white vinegar
- 20 drops tea tree oil (lavender or lemon oil work too)

Directions

1. Pour ingredients into a spray bottle. Spray surfaces and wipe clean.

EATING OUT AT RESTAURANTS

Eating out is convenient but it can feel like a chore if you're trying to navigate a new food plan. Here are my tips for helping you stay on track.

- **Eat a snack before going out to eat.** This can be as simple as a handful of nuts in the car ride over. You won't be as hungry when you arrive and you'll be less tempted by the bread basket.

- **Look at the menu ahead of time and know what you're going to order.** This will take away the stress of figuring it out when you arrive.

- **If options are limited, stick with a salad topped with some type of protein.** Instead of the premade salad dressing, ask for olive oil and vinegar (or lemon wedges).

- **If options are less restricted, stick with meat and vegetable dishes.** Examples: burger wrapped in lettuce with sweet potato fries, roasted salmon with asparagus, dairy-free curries, chicken shawarma with rice, shrimp and vegetable stir fry, any type of customizable bowl with a gluten-free grain, protein and serving of fat (like avocado or tahini dressing).

- **Ask your waiter if you're not sure about the ingredients and describe your food preferences (gluten-free, dairy-free, etc).** They'll point you in the right direction and the kitchen can modify to meet your requests.

- **Take activated charcoal if food quality is ques-tionable.** Activated charcoal binds to any toxic sub-stances and helps flush them out of your body, which makes it beneficial for general detoxification purposes.

MAINTAINING CLEAR SKIN WHILE TRAVELING

Traveling can derail any routine. The following tips can make traveling work in your favor.

- **Pack a meal and snacks for the plane.** This can be something simple like leftover stew in a thermos. If there's good options at the airport, you can pick those up when you arrive. I travel with packets of protein powder, gluten-free oatmeal, beef jerky and stevia.

- **Bring activated charcoal.** You never know when you might need it. In addition to getting rid of toxins from low-quality foods, charcoal also helps get rid of excess gas and bloating, which can occur if you're eat-ing new foods while traveling.

- **Look up restaurants in the area beforehand.** You can filter your search using words like "healthy" or "grass-fed". In terms of cuisine, Mediterranean and Japanese are generally protocol-safe depending on what you order. Mark restaurants that seem like a good fit on your map.

- **Make a run to the grocery store when you first arrive.** You can pick up any snack foods or meals if they have good options at the hot food bar.

- **Let people know what you *can* have, not what you can't**. For example, tell your hosts that you eat most meat and vegetable dishes. That way they can choose restaurants accordingly and grocery shop for the right things. If you need specialty items (like coconut milk) let them know that too.

SUMMARY

Make informed lifestyle choices.

Key takeaways

- Practice five minutes of meditation daily
- Get at least eight hours of sleep every night
- Keep your home free of unnecessary toxins
- Spearmint tea helps with breakouts caused by excess androgens (seen in conditions like polycystic ovarian syndrome)
- For estrogen dominance, consider supplementing with DIM
- At restaurants, look at menus beforehand, stick with meat and vegetable dishes and ask waiters for help
- When traveling, bring easy to pack items like protein powder packets, figure out what your food options are in the area and tell people what you *can* have (not what you can't)

CONCLUSION

When you treat the root causes of acne, rather than suppress it with medications, you restore balance to your inner ecosystem. This allows you to maintain clear skin for the long term.

I hope you're able to take the tools that you've learned from this book and apply them. These tools are now part of your "health tool kit" that you can access at any time. Be your own health detective: be curious, be patient and be willing to experiment. It will all come together.

Now that you have the tools, it's time to put them to use.

CHEAT SHEET

	SAMPLE ROUTINE
7AM	Meditation Breakfast: Mediterranean Chicken Sausage with Artichoke Dip Supplements: multivitamin, omega-3s, digestive enzymes, betaine HCL and supplements specific to your plan
12PM	Workout Water or herbal tea Lunch: Leftovers with Simple Salad and Mustard Vinaigrette Supplements: digestive enzymes and betaine HCL
3PM	Water or herbal tea Snack: nuts
6PM	Water or herbal tea Dinner: Mustard Salmon with Sweet Potato Latkes Supplements: digestive enzymes and betaine HCL

Continued on following page

8PM	Manuka honey cinnamon face mask
	Clean skin routine
10PM	Bed

GUT REPAIR

- 5R framework for gut healing: remove, replace, reinoculate, repair, rebalance
- Don't take antibiotics, acid-blockers, birth control pills or NSAIDs unless medically necessary
- Identify your gut issue—leaky gut, Candida or SIBO—and then follow the treatment plan
- Poop at least 1-2 times daily and drink more water

THERAPEUTIC DIET

- Eat real, whole foods
- Fill half your plate with non-starchy vegetables, one quarter with protein, one quarter with gluten-free grains (or starchy vegetables) and add one serving of fat
- Therapeutic foods for acne: liver and other organ meats, SMASH fish (salmon, mackerel, anchovies, sardines, herring), bone broth, different colored fruits and vegetables, turmeric, green tea, eggs (if allowed on food plan), fermented foods (if allowed on food plan)

- Dairy, sugar, gluten and alcohol are not included in any of the food plans

- Printable versions of the food plans are available on my website, renellestayton.com

- During weeks 1-4, follow your therapeutic food plan

- Starting week 5, begin to reintroduce eliminated foods

- Continue to limit intake of sugar, refined carbohydrates, dairy and alcohol even after the protocol in order to support gut, skin and hormonal health

SUPPLEMENTS

SUPPLEMENT	PLAN	DOSE
Multivitamin, high-quality	All plans (leaky gut, Candida, SIBO)	Take as directed by manufacturer
Omega-3s, fish oil (purified)	All plans	2 grams EPA/DHA daily
Digestive enzymes	All plans	1-2 capsules, with meals
Betaine HCL	All plans, if needed	First, do the baking soda or betaine HCL test. If you do need to take it, take your specific dose with protein-rich meals.

Continued on following page

Probiotics	Leaky gut	10-20 billion CFUs daily Take for one month or longer if needed
L-glutamine	Leaky gut	1-3 grams daily Take for one month or longer if needed
Demulcent herbs (DGL, marshmallow root, slippery elm)	Leaky gut	Take as directed by manufacturer Take for one month or longer if needed Example: GI-Encap by Thorne
Caprylic acid	Candida	800mg twice daily, on an empty stomach Take for one month Example: Caprylic Acid by Pure Encapsulations
Herbal antibiotic blend containing things like berberine, oregano oil and wormwood	SIBO	Dosing depends on product being used Take for one month Example: Candibactin-BR and Candibactin-AR by Metagenics, taken together. Take as directed by the manufacturer.

TOPICAL TREATMENTS

- Choose clean products free from harmful ingredients, use the EWG Skin Deep database
- Use a gentle cleanser with natural, clean ingredients (<10 ingredients ideal)
- Treat with niacinamide (vitamin B3)
- Moisturize with rosehip seed oil, with or without a regular moisturizer
- Optional: diluted apple cider vinegar toner once or twice weekly, aloe vera matcha or manuka honey cinnamon face mask once weekly, mineral makeup
- If you wear makeup, switch to mineral-based makeup and wear it as little as possible

LIFESTYLE HACKS

- Practice five minutes of meditation daily
- Aim for eight hours of sleep every night
- Drink two cups of spearmint tea daily if you suffer from hormonal breakouts related to androgen excess (seen in conditions like polycystic ovarian syndrome)
- For estrogen dominance, consider taking DIM
- Keep your home free of unnecessary toxins
- At restaurants, look at menus beforehand, stick with

meat and vegetable dishes, eat a snack before going out to eat

- While traveling, bring easy to pack items like protein powder packets, figure out what your food options are in the area, tell people what you *can* have (not what you can't)

RECIPES

BEVERAGES
> Bone Broth
>
> Collagen Coffee
>
> Golden Milk
>
> Matcha Latte

BREAKFAST
> AB&J Smoothie
>
> Coconut Cinnamon Smoothie
>
> Mediterranean Chicken Sausage

LUNCH
> Chicken Salad
>
> Coconut Curry Soup

DINNER
> Crispy Garlic Chicken
>
> Mediterranean Platter
>
> Mustard Salmon
>
> Persian Celery Stew (Khoresh-e Karafs)
>
> Thai Meatballs

SIDES

Artichoke Dip

Bacon Brussels Sprouts

Baked Sweet Potatoes

Cauliflower Rice

Guacamole

Mustard Vinaigrette

Quinoa

Roasted Butternut Squash

Simple Salad

Sweet Potato Latkes

DESSERT

Chia Pudding

BEVERAGES

BONE BROTH

Serves: 8

For low-FODMAP: omit onion, garlic and celery

. . . .

Ingredients

- 2 lbs grass-fed beef marrow bones, or any soup bones
- 1 gallon of water
- 2 T apple cider vinegar
- 2 carrots, peeled and cut into rough chunks
- 2 stalks celery, cut into rough chunks
- 1 onion, cut into rough chunks
- 1 clove garlic, smashed (optional)
- Any fresh herbs (optional)
- 1 tsp salt (optional)

Directions

1. In a large stockpot, add the bones, water and apple cider vinegar. Let sit for 20 minutes, allowing the vinegar to extract minerals from the bones.

2. Rough chop the carrot, celery and onion and add it to the pot. Add the salt.

3. Bring the broth to a boil and then reduce to a simmer. Cook over low heat for 24 hours.

4. A frothy layer may form on top as it cooks for the first few hours. Remove this with a spoon.

5. The last 30 minutes of cooking, add the garlic and fresh herbs.

6. Remove from heat and strain using a fine metal strainer or cheesecloth. Store in the refrigerator for up to 4 days and freeze any extra.

TIP: Add all ingredients to the Instant Pot and cook on high pressure for 2 hours. Quick release when it's done.

TIP: Pour the broth into muffin tins and freeze to make bone broth "pucks" that you can use for soup stocks or to drink

COLLAGEN COFFEE

Serves: 1

For Candida: use decaf coffee

. . . .

Ingredients

- 8 oz brewed coffee
- 1 T collagen peptides
- ¼ tsp cinnamon
- Optional: unsweetened non-dairy milk, stevia

Directions

1. Blend all ingredients with a handheld frother or in a blender.

GOLDEN MILK

Serves: 1

. . . .

Ingredients

- 1 cup any unsweetened non-dairy milk (I use almond, coconut or hemp)
- ½ tsp ground turmeric
- ¼ tsp ground ginger (or ½" knob fresh ginger, finely minced)
- ¼ tsp cinnamon
- Pinch of cardamom
- Pinch of black pepper
- Stevia, to taste

Directions

1. Add non-dairy milk and spices to a small saucepan over medium-high heat. Whisk so that spices aren't clumped together.

2. Cover until it comes to a simmer, about 3-5 minutes.

3. Remove from the stove and enjoy.

TIP: You can also buy premade golden milk spice mixes. Just make sure they don't have any added sugars.

MATCHA LATTE

Serves: 1

For Candida: skip this recipe since it's caffeinated

. . . .

Ingredients

- ¾ cup any unsweetened non-dairy milk (I use almond, coconut or hemp)
- ¼ cup hot water (not boiling)
- 1 tsp matcha powder
- Stevia, to taste

Directions

1. Blend matcha and hot water together using a hand frother or bamboo whisk.
2. Add the non-dairy milk and stevia, then blend again.

BREAKFAST

AB&J SMOOTHIE

Serves: 1

For Candida: omit banana

For low-FODMAP: use unripe banana, use strawberries instead of blueberries/blackberries

. . . .

Ingredients

- 1 cup unsweetened non-dairy milk (I use almond, coconut or hemp)
- 1 scoop vanilla protein powder (refer to what protein powder is allowed on your food plan)
- 1 T almond butter
- ½ ripe banana
- ½ cup fresh or frozen blueberries or blackberries
- Handful of spinach or any greens
- Stevia, to taste
- Optional: ice or extra water for thinner consistency

Directions

1. Put all ingredients in a blender and blend until smooth.

COCONUT CINNAMON SMOOTHIE

Serves: 1

. . . .

Ingredients

- ¾ cup coconut milk, full fat, canned (room temperature and well shaken)
- ¼ cup bone broth
- 2 T vanilla protein powder (refer to what protein powder is allowed on your food plan)
- ½ tsp cinnamon
- Stevia, to taste
- Optional: ice or extra water for thinner consistency

Directions

1. Put all ingredients in a blender. Blend on high for 1-2 minutes until coconut milk isn't separated and consistency is smooth.

TIP: Buy bone broth to save time. I use chicken bone broth for this recipe.

MEDITERRANEAN CHICKEN SAUSAGE

Makes: 10 small patties

. . . .

Ingredients

- 1 lb ground chicken thighs
- 1 cup cooked brown rice
- 1T Za'atar spice
- ¼ cup pitted Kalamata olives, diced
- ¼ cup green onion, chopped (green tops only for low-FODMAP)
- ¼ cup parsley, chopped
- ½ tsp salt
- ½ tsp ghee

Directions

1. Add all of the ingredients (except ghee) to a large bowl and mix well.

2. Heat a skillet over medium-high heat and lightly coat the pan with ghee.

3. Take ¼ scoops of the chicken and flatten into patties. Cook for 4-5 minutes per side or until golden brown.

4. Serve with artichoke dip (see recipe under Sides).

TIP: Make this and the artichoke dip on meal prep day so you'll have breakfast for the entire week.

LUNCH

CHICKEN SALAD

Serves: 8

For low-FODMAP: omit celery

. . . .

Ingredients

- 1 rotisserie chicken, shredded
- 4 stalks celery, diced
- ½ cup egg-free mayo (look for vegan brands)
- ½ cup mustard vinaigrette (recipe under Sides)
- 2 T parsley or any fresh herbs

Directions

1. Add all ingredients to a large bowl and mix well.
2. Serve on top of a salad or gluten-free toast. Store in the refrigerator for up to 3 days.

COCONUT CURRY SOUP

Serves: 4

For leaky gut: use shrimp instead of tofu (pan fry shrimp before adding it to the soup at the end)

For Candida: use 1 delicata squash and 1 rutabaga instead of acorn squash and potatoes

. . . .

Ingredients

- 1 (13.5 oz) can unsweetened full fat coconut milk
- 1½ cups water
- 2 carrots, peeled and cut into ½" slices
- 1 acorn squash, halved, seeded and cut into ½" slices
- 2 red potatoes, peeled and cut into 1" cubes
- 1 zucchini, sliced
- 1" chunk fresh ginger, peeled and minced
- Juice of ½ lime
- 2 tsp turmeric
- 1 tsp cumin
- 2 tsp salt
- ½ tsp ghee
- 1 cup firm tofu, cubed
- Optional: cilantro and/or pumpkin seeds for garnish

Directions

1. Prepare all of your vegetables. Set aside.

2. In a large soup pot, heat up ghee over medium heat. Add ginger and cook for 5 minutes until soft. Then add turmeric and cumin, cook for 30 seconds.

3. Add all of the vegetables to the pot and stir to coat them in the spices.

4. Add the coconut milk, water and salt. Scrape off any browned bits from the bottom of the pot. Once boiling, reduce to a simmer.

5. Cover and cook for 20 minutes (until the potatoes are soft). Add the cubed tofu during the last five minutes of cooking.

6. Remove from heat and stir in the lime juice. For a thicker, creamier soup, take out 1 cup of the soup and blend it on high, then stir it back into the soup.

7. Garnish with fresh cilantro and pumpkin seeds before serving.

TIP: To make this vegan-friendly, substitute coconut oil for ghee.

DINNER

CRISPY GARLIC CHICKEN

Serves: 6

For low-FODMAP: avoid this recipe because it contains a lot of garlic

. . . .

Ingredients

- 2 lbs boneless, skinless chicken thighs
- 8 large cloves garlic, minced (use a garlic press if you have it)
- 1 T dry white wine (such as Sauvignon blanc)
- 1 T dried oregano
- 1 tsp salt

Directions

1. Preheat the oven to 350°F.
2. Place chicken in a shallow baking dish.
3. Pour the white wine over the chicken. Sprinkle the oregano and salt on top, then spread the minced garlic over the chicken so that it's evenly coated.
4. Bake for 30-35 minutes until the garlic is crispy and the chicken is lightly browned and cooked through.

MEDITERRANEAN PLATTER

Serves: 4

For low-FODMAP: instead of the chicken and marinade use plain rotisserie chicken, look for hummus without garlic

. . . .

Ingredients

- 1 cucumber, cut into sticks for dipping (about 3" long)
- 1 bag baby carrots
- 2 large tomatoes, sliced
- 1 bunch of basil
- 14 oz can artichoke hearts (packed in water), drained and sliced in half
- ½ cup Kalamata olives, pitted
- Hummus (10 oz tub), dairy-free
- Optional: dolmas or falafels

For the chicken and marinade

1. 2 lbs boneless, skinless chicken thighs
2. Juice of 1 lemon
3. 10 cloves garlic, minced
4. 1 T fresh thyme
5. Salt to taste

Directions

1. Marinate the chicken in the lemon juice, garlic, thyme and salt for at least 30 minutes before making.

2. Turn the grill to medium high heat. Grill the chicken until the internal temperature reaches 135°F (about 7-8 minutes per side). Remove from heat and let it sit for at least 3-5 minutes before cutting.

3. Prep your vegetables after you're done cooking the chicken. Then, divide the platter ingredients evenly amongst four plates. I like to put the hummus in the middle and spread the rest of the ingredients around it.

TIP: To make this vegetarian or vegan-friendly, substitute falafel for chicken. Just make sure the ingredients work with your food plan.

MUSTARD SALMON

Serves: 4

. . . .

Ingredients

- 4 salmon fillets, skin on (about 6 oz each)
- ¼ cup Dijon mustard
- ¼ cup parsley, chopped
- Juice of ½ lemon
- Pinch of salt and pepper

Directions

1. Preheat oven to 375°F. Line a baking sheet with parchment paper.

2. In a small bowl, mix together Dijon, lemon juice and parsley. Set aside.

3. Pat each salmon fillet dry and place salmon skin side down on the baking sheet. Season with salt and pepper.

4. Take 1 tablespoon of Dijon mixture and spread on top of each salmon fillet.

5. Bake for 12-15 minutes until salmon is cooked through. Let sit for 10 minutes before serving.

PERSIAN CELERY STEW (KHORESH-E KARAFS)

Serves: 8

For low-FODMAP: avoid this recipe because it contains a lot of celery, garlic and onions

. . . .

Ingredients

- 2 lbs lamb stew meat
- 2 cups water
- 2 heads celery, cut into 1" pieces
- 2 bunches of flat leaf parsley, finely chopped
- 1 bunch of fresh mint, finely chopped (or 1 T dried mint)
- 1 large yellow onion, diced
- 2 cloves garlic, minced
- ¼ cup lime juice (about 2 limes)
- 2 tsp salt
- 2 tsp turmeric
- ½ tsp saffron, dissolved in 2 T hot water
- ½ tsp ghee

Directions

1. In a large soup pot, sauté onion in ghee until it's soft and translucent, about 5 minutes.

2. Add stew meat and garlic, stirring occasionally until the meat is browned.

3. Add the rest of the ingredients to the pot and bring to a boil.

4. Reduce to a simmer, cover and cook for 2 hours.

5. Adjust seasoning to taste and serve.

TIP: Make this in the Instant Pot. Follow the same directions from the beginning, using the sauté button. Once the meat is browned and you're ready to add the rest of the ingredients, the only modification is to use 1½ cups of water instead of 2. Secure the lid and hit the meat/stew button, set the time for 20 minutes. When it's finished, let it naturally release (takes about 20 minutes).

THAI MEATBALLS

Makes: 12 meatballs

. . . .

Ingredients

- 1 lb ground beef
- ¼ cup green onion, chopped (green tops only for low-FODMAP)
- ¼ cup cilantro, chopped
- 1 large carrot, finely shredded
- 1 T fresh ginger, peeled and minced
- 1 tsp salt

Sauce

- ¼ cup coconut aminos
- 1 T fish sauce (optional)
- 1 T toasted sesame oil
- 1 T fresh ginger, peeled and minced

Directions

1. Preheat oven to 400°F. Line a baking sheet with parchment paper.
2. In a medium-sized bowl, mix together the ground beef, green onion, cilantro, carrot, ginger and salt.

3. Use a cookie scooper (or your hands) to scoop out meatballs and put them on the baking sheet. Bake for 20-25 minutes, until meatballs are browned.

4. Prepare your sauce while the meatballs are baking. In a small bowl, whisk together the sauce ingredients. When the meatballs are done, drizzle the sauce on top.

5. Serve meatballs with rice and steamed baby bok choy.

TIP: Double the meatball recipe and freeze the second batch so you can use it for a quick meal.

FOR RICE AND BABY BOK CHOY: Before making the meatballs, start cooking a cup of brown rice (follow directions on bag) or use leftover brown rice. Start steaming the baby bok choy 10 minutes before the meatballs come out of the oven. Add 1" of water to a large pot with a steaming basket. Put over medium-high heat. Once simmering, add bok choy to the basket. Steam for about 7 min, until bright green and base is tender.

SIDES

ARTICHOKE DIP

. . . .

Ingredients

- 1 (14 oz) can artichoke hearts, drained
- ⅓ cup extra virgin olive oil
- Juice of 1 small lemon
- 2 T tahini
- 1½ tsp turmeric
- Pinch of cayenne (optional)
- ½ tsp salt

Directions

1. Add all ingredients to a high speed blender and blend until smooth.

BACON BRUSSELS SPROUTS

Serves: 4

For low-FODMAP: avoid this recipe because it contains Brussels sprouts

. . . .

Ingredients

- 1 lb Brussels sprouts
- 3 slices nitrite-free bacon, chopped into small pieces
- 2 T ghee, melted
- Salt and pepper, to taste

Directions

1. Preheat oven to 400°F. Line a baking sheet with parchment paper.

2. Trim the ends and any old leaves off of the Brussels sprouts, then cut them in half.

3. Toss the Brussels sprouts with melted ghee and bacon pieces. Spread it evenly over the baking sheet. Season with a pinch of salt and pepper.

4. Bake for 30-35 minutes, until Brussels sprouts are crispy and browned.

BAKED SWEET POTATOES

For low-FODMAP: limit serving to ½ cup

. . . .

Ingredients

- 4 small sweet potatoes

Directions

1. Preheat oven to 400°F. Line a baking sheet with parchment paper

2. Wash the sweet potatoes and then poke a few holes in each with a knife or fork (allows steam to release while baking).

3. Arrange sweet potatoes on the baking sheet a few inches apart. Bake for 45 minutes to 1 hour, or until sweet potatoes are tender.

TIP: To make these in the Instant Pot, put 1" of water and the steam rack inside the pot. Hit the "manual/pressure cook" button and set to high pressure for 15 minutes. Let it quick release.

CAULIFLOWER RICE

For low-FODMAP: avoid this recipe
because it contains cauliflower

. . . .

Ingredients

- 1 medium head of cauliflower, roughly chopped into medium-sized chunks
- ½ tsp coconut oil
- Salt, to taste

Directions

1. Add cauliflower chunks to a blender or food processor, about 2 cups at a time. Pulse until rice-like consistency. (You may have to scrape the edges frequently to make sure all of the pieces are riced).

2. In a large skillet, heat coconut oil over medium-high heat. Add riced cauliflower. Cover and cook for about 5-7 minutes, until cauliflower is soft but not mushy. Season with salt.

TIP: Buy pre-riced cauliflower. You can find this in the fresh or frozen produce section.

GUACAMOLE

Serves: 2

For low-FODMAP: avoid this recipe because
it contains a lot of avocados, onions and garlic

. . . .

Ingredients

- 2 avocados, ripe
- ¼ cup salsa
- Juice of 1 lime
- Salt and pepper, to taste

Directions

1. Peel and mash avocado in a medium sized bowl. Add
   salsa, lime juice, salt and pepper. Mix well to incorporate.

MUSTARD VINAIGRETTE

. . . .

Ingredients

- ¾ cup extra virgin olive oil
- 2 T apple cider vinegar
- Juice of 1 lemon
- 2 tsp Dijon mustard
- ½ tsp salt
- 2 drops liquid stevia

Directions

1. Add all ingredients to the blender and blend.
2. Adjust seasoning as desired.

QUINOA

Makes: 3 cups cooked quinoa

. . . .

Ingredients

- 1 cup quinoa, rinsed and drained
- 2 cups water (or bone broth)
- ¼ tsp salt

Directions

1. Add all ingredients to a medium sized saucepan.
2. Bring to a boil, then reduce to keep at a low simmer. Cook uncovered for 15-20 minutes, until all of the water is absorbed. Remove from heat and cover for 5 minutes.
3. Fluff with a fork before serving

ROASTED BUTTERNUT SQUASH

Serves: 8

For Candida: avoid this recipe as butternut squash is a starchy vegetable

For low-FODMAP: limit serving to ¼ cup

. . . .

Ingredients

- 1 butternut squash, halved, peeled, seeded and chopped into 1-2" pieces
- 2 T ghee, melted
- Salt and pepper, to taste

Directions

1. Preheat oven to 400°F. Line a baking sheet with parchment paper.
2. Toss butternut squash with melted ghee, salt and pepper. Spread evenly over baking sheet.
3. Bake for 40 minutes, until browned.

TIP: Buy butternut squash that's already been prepped.

SIMPLE SALAD

Serves: 2

. . . .

Ingredients

- 4 handfuls of any salad greens
- 1 large carrot, shredded
- ¼ large cucumber, halved and sliced thin
- Any other toppings you want: avocado, radishes, pumpkin seeds, etc.

Directions

1. Mix all of the ingredients in a large salad bowl.

SWEET POTATO LATKES

Makes: 8 latkes

For Candida: avoid this recipe because it contains sweet potatoes and arrowroot which are starchy

For low-FODMAP: avoid this recipe because it contains coconut flour

. . . .

Ingredients

- 2 cups peeled and shredded Japanese sweet potato (about 1 large sweet potato, use biggest grating size)
- ¼ cup coconut flour
- ¼ cup arrowroot powder
- ¼ cup green onions, chopped (green tops only for low-FODMAP)
- Juice of ½ a lemon
- ½ tsp salt
- 2 tsp ghee

Directions

1. Peel and shred the sweet potato. Put shreddings in a clean towel and wring out as much excess liquid as possible.

2. In a medium-sized bowl, mix together the coconut

flour, arrowroot and salt.

3. Add the sweet potato shreddings, green onion and lemon juice. Mix well with your hands to combine.

4. Heat a skillet over medium-high heat and add ghee.

5. Add ¼ cup scoops of the latke mixture to the skillet and flatten with a spatula. Cook about 5-6 minutes per side, or until golden brown.

DESSERT

CHIA PUDDING

. . . .

Ingredients

- ½ cup chia seeds
- 3 cups any non-dairy milk
- 1 tsp vanilla extract
- 2 tsp cocoa powder (optional)
- Stevia, to taste

Directions

1. Add all ingredients to a bowl and stir well.
2. Cover and put in the refrigerator. Let it sit for at least 2 hours before serving, giving it another good stir after 1 hour.
3. Add more milk if the pudding is too thick or more chia seeds if it's too runny.

REFERENCES

WHY YOU HAVE ACNE

1. Taniguchi K, Karin M. IL-6 and related cytokines as the critical lynchpins between inflammation and cancer. *Semin Immunol.* 2014 Feb;26(1):54-74.
2. Lontchi-Yimagou E, Sobngwi E, Matsha TE, et al. Diabetes mellitus and inflammation. *Curr Diab Rep.* 2013 Jun;13(3):435-44.
3. Golia E, Limongelli G, Natale F, et al. Inflammation and cardiovascular disease: from pathogenesis to therapeutic target. *Curr Atheroscler Rep.* 2014 Sept;16(9):435.
4. Miller AH, Maletic V, Raison CL. Inflammation and its discontents: the role of cytokines in the pathophysiology of major depression. *Biol Psychiatry.* 2009 May 1;65(9):732-41.
5. Chitnis T, Weiner HL. CNS inflammation and neurodegeneration. *J Clin Invest.* 2017 Oct 2;127(10):3577-87.
6. Tanghetti EA. The role of inflammation in the pathology of acne. *J Clin Aesthet Dermatol.* 2013 Sep;6(9):27-35.
7. Jeremy AH, Holland DB, Roberts SG, et al. Inflammatory events are involved in acne lesion initiation. *J Invest Dermatol.* 2003 Jul;121(1):20-27.
8. Ingham E, Eady EA, Goodwin CE, et al. Pro-inflammatory levels of interleukin-1 alpha-like bioactivity are present in the majority of open comedones in acne vulgaris. *J Invest Dermatol.* 1992 Jun;98(6):895-901.
9. Kucharska A, Szmurło A, Sińska B. Significance of diet in treated and untreated acne vulgaris. *Postepy Dermatol Alergol.* 2016 Apr;33(2):81-86.

10. Bowe WP, Joshi SS, Shalita AR. Diet and acne. *J Am Acad Dermatol.* 2010 Jul;63(1):124-141.

11. Çerman AA, Aktaş E, Altunay K, et al. Dietary glycemic factors, insulin resistance, and adiponectin levels in acne vulgaris. *J Am Acad Dermatol.* 2016 Jul;75(1):155-162.

12. Smith RN, Mann NJ, Braue A, et al. The effect of a high-protein, low glycemic-load diet versus a conventional high glycemic-load diet on biochemical parameters associated with acne vulgaris: a randomized, investigator-masked, controlled trial. *J Am Acad Dermatol.* 2007 Aug;57(2):247-256.

13. Kwon HH, Yoon JY, Hong JS, et al. Clinical and histological effect of a low glycemic load diet in treatment of acne vulgaris in Korean patients: a randomized, controlled trial. *Acta Derm Venereol.* 2012 May;92(3):241-246.

14. Ismail NH, Manaf ZA, Azizan NZ. High glycemic load diet, milk and ice cream consumption are related to acne in Malaysian young adults: a case control study. *BMC Dermatol.* 2012 Aug 16;12:13.

15. Juhl CR, Bergholdt HKM, Miller IM, et al. Dairy intake and acne vulgaris: a systematic review and meta-analysis of 78,529 children, adolescents and young adults. *Nutrients.* 2018 Aug 9;10(8).

16. Melnik BC. Evidence for acne-promoting effects of milk and other insulinotropic dairy products. *Nestle Nutr Workshop Ser Pediatr Program.* 2011;67:131-145.

17. Norat T, Dossus L, Rinaldi S, et al. Diet, serum insulin-like growth factor-1 and IGF-binding protein-3 in European women. *Eur J Clin Nutr.* 2007 Jan;61(1):91-98.

18. Melnik BC, Schmitz G. Role of insulin, insulin-like growth factor-1, hyperglycaemic food and milk consumption in the pathogenesis of acne vulgaris. *Experimental Dermatology.* 2009 Oct;18(10):833-841.

19. Hoppe C, Mølgaard C, Dalum C, et al. Differential effects of casein versus whey on fasting plasma levels of insulin, IGF-1 and IGF-1/IGFBP-3: results from a randomized 7-day supplementation study in prepubertal boys. *Eur J Clin Nutr.* 2009;63:1076-1083.

20. Lee YB, Byun EJ, Kim HS. Potential role of the microbiome in acne: A comprehensive review. *J Clin Med.* 2019 Jul;8(7):987.

21. Mu Quinghui, Kirby J, Reilly CM, et al. Leaky gut as a danger signal

for autoimmune diseases. *Front Immunol.* 2017;8:598.

22. Sturgeon C, Fasano A. Zonulin, a regulator of epithelial and endo-thelial barrier functions, and its involvement in chronic inflammatory diseases. *Tissue Barriers.* 2016 Oct 21;4(4):e1251384.

23. Hollon J, Puppa EL, Greenwald B, et al. Effect of gliadin on permeabil-ity of intestinal biopsy explants from celiac disease patients and patients with non-celiac gluten sensitivity. *Nutrients.* 2015 Mar;7(3):1565-1576.

24. Konturek PC, Brzozowski T, Konturek SJ. Stress and the gut: patho-physiology, clinical consequences, diagnostic approach and treatment options. *Journal of Physiology and Pharmacology.* 2011 Dec;62(6):591-599.

25. Yang X, Li Y, Li Y, et al. Oxidative stress-mediated atherosclerosis: mechanisms and therapies. *Front Physiol.* 2017;8:600.

26. De Rosa S, Cirillo P, Paglia A, et al. Reactive oxygen species and an-tioxidants in the pathophysiology of cardiovascular disease: does the actual knowledge justify a clinical approach? *Curr Vasc Pharmacol.* 2010 Mar; 8(2):259-75.

27. Ullah A, Khan A, Khan I. Diabetes mellitus and oxidative stress-a con-cise review. *Saudi Pharmaceutical Journal.* 2016 Sep;24(5):547-53.

28. Domej W, Oettl K, Renner W. Oxidative stress and free radicals in COPD-implications and relevance for treatment. *Int J Chron Obstruct Pulm Dis.* 2014 Oct 17;9:1207-24.

29. Smallwood MJ, Nissim A, Knight AR, et al. Oxidative stress in auto-immune rheumatic diseases. *Free Radical Biology and Medicine.* 2018 Sep;125:3-14.

30. Sahib AS, Al-Anbari HH, Raghif AR. Oxidative stress in acne vulgar-is: an important therapeutic target. *Journal of Molecular Pathophysiology.* 2013 April 1;2:27-31.

31. Sarici G, Cinar S, Armutcu F, et al. Oxidative stress in acne vulgaris. *J Eur Acad Dermatol Venereol.* 2010 July;24(7):763-7.

32. Jówko E, Różański P, Tomczak A. Effects of a 36-h survival train-ing with sleep deprivation on oxidative stress and muscle damage bio-markers in young healthy men. *Int J Environ Res Public Health.* 2018 Oct;15(10):2066.

GUT REPAIR

1. Chedid V, Dhalla S, Clarke JO, et al. Herbal therapy is equivalent to rifaximin for the treatment of small intestinal bacterial overgrowth. *Glob Adv Health Med.* 2014 May;3(3):16-24.
2. Miyano Y, Sakata I, Kuroda K, et al. The role of the vagus nerve in the migrating motor complex and ghrelin- and motilin-induced gastric contraction in suncus. *PLoS ONE.* 2013 May;8(5):e64777.
3. Pimentel M, Soffer EE, Chow EJ, et al. Lower frequency of MMC is found in IBS subjects with abnormal lactulose breath test, suggesting bacterial overgrowth. *Digestive Diseases and Sciences.* 2002;47:2639-2643.

THERAPEUTIC DIET

1. Ozuguz P, Kacar SD, Ekiz O, et al. Evaluation of serum vitamins A and E and zinc levels according to severity of acne vulgaris. *Cutan Ocul Toxicol.* 2014 June;33(2):99-102.
2. Gaber HA, Abozied AA, Abd-Elkareem IM, et al. Serum zinc levels in patients with acne vulgaris and its relation to the severity of disease. *The Egyptian Journal of Hospital Medicine.* 2019,75(5):2845-2848.
3. Michaëlsson G, Ljunghall K. Patients with dermatitis herpetiformis, acne, psoriasis and Darier's disease have low epidermal zinc concentrations. *Acta Derm Venereol.* 1990;70(4):304-308.
4. El-Akawi Z, Abdel-Latif N, Abdul-Razzak K. Does the plasma level of vitamins A and E affect acne condition? *Clin Exp Dermatol.* 2006 May;31(3):430-434.
5. Daley CA, Abbot A, Doyle PS, et al. A review of fatty acid profiles and antioxidant content in grass-fed and grain-fed beef. *Nutrition Journal.* 2010 March 10;9:10.
6. Crinnion WJ. Organic foods contain higher levels of certain nutrients, lower levels of pesticides, and may provide health benefits for the consumer. *Altern Med Rev.* 2010 Apr;15(1):4-12.
7. Lu C, Barr DB, Pearson MA, et al. Dietary intake and its contribution to longitudinal organophosphorus pesticide exposure in urban/subur-

ban children. *Environ Health Perspect.* 2008 Apr;116(4):537-542.

8. Lu C, Toepel K, Irish R, et al. Organic diets significantly lower children's dietary exposure to organophosphorus pesticides. *Environ Health Perspect.* 2006 Feb;114(2):260-263.

9. Rull RP, Ritz B, Shaw GM. Neural tube defects and maternal residential proximity to agricultural pesticide applications. *Am J Epidemiol.* 2006 Apr 15;163(8):743-53.

10. Garry VF, Harkins ME, Erickson LL, et al. Birth defects, season of conception, and sex of children born to pesticide applicators living in the Red River Valley of Minnesota, USA. *Environ Health Perspect.* 2002 Jun;110(Suppl 3):441-449.

11. Zhang L, Rana I, Shaffer RM, et al. Exposure to glyphosate-based herbicides and risk for non-Hodgkin lymphoma: A meta-analysis and supporting evidence. *Mutat Res.* 2019 Feb 10;781:186-206.

12. Sanin LH, Carrasquilla G, Solomon KR, et al. Regional differences in time to pregnancy among fertil women from five Columbian regions with different use of glyphosate. *J Toxicol Environ Health A.* 2009;72(15-16):949-60.

13. Panahi Y, Darvishi B, Ghanei M, et al. Molecular mechanisms of curcumins suppressing effects on tumorigenesis, angiogenesis and metastasis, focusing on NF-kB pathway. *Cytokine Growth Factor Rev.* 2016 Apr;28:21-29.

14. Saric S, Notay M, Sivamani RK. Green tea and other tea polyphenols: effects on sebum production and acne vulgaris. *Antioxidants (Basel).* 2017 Mar;6(1):2.

15. Katiyar SK, Ahmad N, Mukhtar H. Green tea and skin. *Arch Dermatol.* 2000 Aug;136(8)989-994.

16. Katiyar SK, Elmets CA, Agarwal R, et al. Protection against ultraviolet-B radiation-induced local and systemic suppression of contact hypersensitivity and edema responses in C3H/HeN mice by green tea polyphenols. *Photochem Photobiol.* 1995 Nov;62(5):855-861.

17. Oyetakin White P, Tribout H, Baron E. Protective mechanisms of green tea polyphenols in skin. *Oxid Med Cell Longev.* 2012;2012:560682.

18. Yoon JY, Kwon HH, Min SU, et al. Epigallocatechin-3-gallate improves acne in humans by modulating intracellular targets and inhibiting P. acnes. *J Invest Dermatol.* 2013 Feb;133(2):429-440.

19. Weiss DJ, Anderton CR. Determination of catechins in matcha green tea by micellar electrokinetic chromatography. *J Chromatogr A.* 2003 Sep 5;1011(1-2):173-180.

20. Karsten HD, Patterson PH, Stout R, et al. Vitamins A, E and fatty acid composition of the eggs of caged hens and pastured hens. *Renewable Agriculture and Food Systems.* 2010 Jan 12;25(1):45-54.

21. Sturgeon C, Fasano A. Zonulin, a regulator of epithelial and endothelial barrier functions, and its involvement in chronic inflammatory diseases. *Tissue Barriers.* 2016 Oct 21;4(4):e1251384.

22. Hollon J, Puppa EL, Greenwald B, et al. Effect of gliadin on permeability of intestinal biopsy explants from celiac disease patients and patients with non-celiac gluten sensitivity. *Nutrients.* 2015 Mar;7(3):1565-1576.

SUPPLEMENTS

1. Ozuguz P, Kacar SD, Ekiz O, et al. Evaluation of serum vitamins A and E and zinc levels according to severity of acne vulgaris. *Cutan Ocul Toxicol.* 2014 June;33(2):99-102.

2. Gaber HA, Abozied AA, Abd-Elkareem IM, et al. Serum zinc levels in patients with acne vulgaris and its relation to the severity of disease. *The Egyptian Journal of Hospital Medicine.* 2019,75(5):2845-2848.

3. Michaëlsson G, Ljunghall K. Patients with dermatitis herpetiformis, acne, psoriasis and Darier's disease have low epidermal zinc concentrations. *Acta Derm Venereol.* 1990;70(4):304-308.

4. Michaëlsson G, Juhlin L, Ljunghall K. A double-blind study of the effect of zinc and oxytetracycline in acne vulgaris. *Br J Dermatol.* 1977 Nov;97(5):561-566.

5. Calder PC. Omega-3 fatty acids and inflammatory processes: from molecules to man. *Biochem Soc Trans.* 2017 Oct 15;45(5):1105-1115.

6. Jung JY, Kwon HH, Hong JS, et al. Effect of dietary supplementation with omega-3 fatty acid and gamma-linolenic acid on acne vulgaris: a randomized, double-blind, controlled trial. *Acta Derm Venereol.* 2014 Sep;94(5):521-525.

7. Yeşilova Y, Çalka Ö, Akdeniz N, et al. Effect of probiotics on the

treatment of children with atopic dermatitis. *Annals of Dermatology.* 2012;24(2):189–93.

8. Kim J, Ko Y, Park YK, et al. Dietary effect of lactoferrin-enriched fermented milk on skin surface lipid and clinical improvement of acne vulgaris. *Nutrition.* 2010;26:902–9.

9. Hacini-Rachinel F, Gheit H, Le Luduec JB, et al. Oral probiotic control skin inflammation by acting on both effector and regulatory T cells. *PLoS ONE.* 2009;4(3):e4903.

10. Gueniche A, Philippe D, Bastien P, et al. Randomised double-blind placebo-controlled study of the effect of Lactobacillus paracasei NCC 2461 on skin reactivity. *Benef Microbes.* 2013;5:137–45.

11. Yan HM, Zhao HJ, Guo DY, et al. Gut microbiota alterations in moderate to severe acne vulgaris patients. *J Dermatol.* 2018 Oct;45(10):1166-1171.

12. Deng Y, Wang H, Zhou J, et al. Patients with acne vulgaris have distinct gut microbiota in comparison with healthy controls. *Acta Derm Venereol.* 2018 Aug 29;98(8):783-790.

13. Rao RK, Samak G. Role of glutamine in protection of intestinal epithelial tight junctions. *J Epithel Biol Pharmacol.* 2011;5(Suppl1-M7):47-54.

14. Bakovic M. The roles of glutamine in the intestine and its implication in intestinal diseases. *Int J Mol Sci.* 2017 May;18(5):1051.

15. Chedid V, Dhalla S, Clarke JO, et al. Herbal therapy is equivalent to rifaximin for the treatment of small intestinal bacterial overgrowth. *Glob Adv Health Med.* 2014 May;3(3):16-24.

16. Lan J, Zhao Y, Dong F, et al. Meta-analysis of the effect and safety of berberine in the treatment of type 2 diabetes mellitus, hyperlipidemia and hypertension. *J Ethnopharmacol.* 2015 Feb 23;161:69-81.

17. Tew XN, Lau NJ, Chellappan DK, et al. Immunological axis of berberine in managing inflammation underlying chronic respiratory inflammatory diseases. *Chem Biol Interact.* 2020 Jan 20;317:108947.

18. Acila-Lozano CC, Loarca-Piña G, Lecona-Uribe S, et al. Oregano: Properties, composition and biological activity. *Arch Latinoam Nutr.* 2004 Mar;54(1):100-111.

19. Juteau F, Jerkovic I, Masotti V, et al. Composition and antimicrobial activity of the essential oil of Artemisia absinthium from Croatia and France. *Planta Med.* 2003;69(2):158-161.

TOPICAL TREATMENTS

1. Bilal M, Iqbal HMN. An insight into toxicity and human-health-related adverse consequences of cosmeceuticals-a review. *Sci Total Environ.* 2019 Jun 20;670:555-568.

2. Pan S, Yuan C, Tagmount A, et al. Parabens and human epidermal growth factor receptor ligand cross-talk in breast cancer cells. *Environmental Health Perspectives.* 2016 May 1; 124(5).

3. Weatherly LM, Gosse JA. Triclosan exposure, transformation, and human health effects. *J Toxicol Environ Health B Crit Rev.* 2018 Sep 6;20(8):447-469.

4. Garg T, Ramam M, Parischa JS, et al. Long term topical application of lactic acid/lactate lotion as a preventative treatment for acne vulgaris. *Indian J Dermatol Venereol Leprol.* 2002 May-Jun;68(3):137-139.

5. Bae JY, Park SN. Evaluation of anti-microbial activities of ZnO, citric acid and a mixture of both against Propionibacterium acnes. *Int J Cosmet Sci.* 2016 Dec;38(6):550-557.

6. Sachdeva S. Lactic acid peeling superficial acne scarring in Indian skin. *J Cosmet Dermatol.* 2010 Sep;9(3):246-248.

7. Wang Y, Kuo S, Shu M, et al. Staphylococcus epidermidis in the human skin microbiome mediates fermentation to inhibit growth of Propionibacterium acnes: implications of probiotics in acne vulgaris. *Appl Microbiol Biotechnol.* 2014 Jan;98(1):411-424.

8. Draelos ZD, Matsubara A, Smiles, K. The effect of 2% niacinamide on facial sebum production. *Journal of Cosmetic and Laser Therapy.* 2006;8(2):96-101.

9. Niren, NM. Pharmacologic doses of nicotinamide in the treatment of inflammatory skin conditions: a review. *Cutis.* 2006 Jan;77(1 Suppl):11-6.

10. Shalita AR, Smith JG, Parish LC, et al. Topical nicotinamide compared with clindamycin gel in the treatment of inflammatory acne vulgaris. *Int J Dermatol.* 1995 Jun;34(6):434-437.

11. Khodaeiani E, Fouladi RF, Amirnia M, et al. Topical 4% nicotinamide vs 1% clindamycin in moderate inflammatory acne vulgaris. *International Journal of Dermatology.* 2013;52(8):999-1004.

12. Downing DT, Stewart ME, Wertz PW, et al. Essential fatty acids and

acne. *J Am Acad Dermatol.* 1986 Feb;14(2 Pt 1):221-225.

13. Oláh A, Tóth B, Borbíró I, et al. Cannabidiol exerts sebostatic and antiinflammatory effects on human sebocytes. *J Clin Invest.* 2014 Sep 2;124(9):3713-3724.

14. Mahmood T, Akhtar N, Khan BA, et al. Outcomes of 3% green tea emulsion on skin sebum production in male volunteers. *Bosn J Basic Med Sci.* 2010 Aug;10(3):260-264.

15. Elsaie ML, Abdelhamid MF, Elsaaiee LT, et al. The efficacy of topical 2% green tea lotion in mild-to-moderate acne vulgaris. *J Drugs Dermatol.* 2009 Apr;8(4):358-364.

16. Hong YH, Jung EY, Shin KS, et al. Tannase-converted green tea catechins and their anti-wrinkle activity in humans. *J Cosmet Dermatol.* 2013 Jun;12(2):137-143.

17. Julianti E, Rajah KK, Fidrianny I. Antibacterial activity of ethanolic extract of cinnamon bark, honey, and their combination effects against acne-causing bacteria. *Sci Pharm.* 2017 Apr 11;85(2):19.

18. Vasconcelos NG, Croda J, Simionatto S. Antibacterial mechanisms of cinnamon and its constituents: a review. *Microb Pathog.* 2018 Jul;120:198-203.

LIFESTYLE HACKS

1. Desbordes G, Negi LT, Pace TWW, et al. Effects of mindful-attention and compassion meditation training on amygdala response to emotional stimuli in an ordinary, non-meditative state. *Front Hum Neurosci.* 2012 Nov;6:292.

2. Grant P. Spearmint herbal tea has significant anti-androgen effects in polycystic ovarian syndrome. *Phytother Res.* 2010 Feb;24(2):186-8.

3. Akdoğan M, Tamer MN, Cüre E, et al. Effect of spearmint (mentha spicata labiatae) teas on androgen levels in women with hirsutism. *Phytother Res.* 2007 May;21(5):444-447.

ABOUT THE AUTHOR

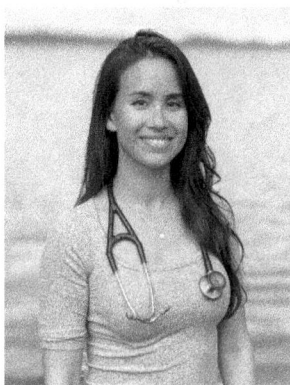

Renelle Stayton is a functional medicine nurse practitioner and holistic nutritionist in Victoria, British Columbia. Trained at the University of California, San Francisco and the Institute for Functional Medicine, her approach is to treat the root causes of problems, not just the symptoms. Using food as medicine and helping people treat chronic skin conditions like acne are her personal areas of interest. She enjoys playing the ukulele, baking healthy desserts and spending time outdoors with her family. To find out more about Renelle's writings, videos and recipes, visit RenelleStayton.com.